THE
NATURAL
TESTOSTERONE
PLAN

THE
NATURAL
TESTOSTERONE
PLAN

FOR SEXUAL HEALTH AND ENERGY

Stephen Harrod Buhner

Healing Arts Press
Rochester, Vermont

Healing Arts Press
One Park Street
Rochester, Vermont 05767
www.HealingArtsPress.com

Healing Arts Press is a division of Inner Traditions International

*Note to the reader: This book is intended as an informational guide. The remedies,
approaches, and techniques described herein are meant to supplement, and not to
be a substitute for, professional medical care or treatment. They should not be used
to treat a serious ailment without prior consultation with a qualified health care
professional.*

Library of Congress Cataloging-in-Publication Data
Buhner, Stephen Harrod.
  The natural testosterone plan : for sexual health and energy / Stephen Harrod
Buhner.
    p. cm.
  Includes bibliographical references and index
  ISBN-13: 978-1-59477-168-2 (alk. paper)
  ISBN-10: 1-59477-168-5 (alk. paper)
  1. Testosterone—Physiological effect. 2. Testosterone—Therapeutic use. I. Title.
  QP572.T4B84 2007
  615'.366—dc22
                                                                    2007001169
Printed and bound in Canada by Transcontinental

10 9 8 7 6 5 4 3 2 1

Text design and layout by Jon Desautels
This book was typeset in Sabon with Futura used as the display typeface

To send correspondence to the author of this book, mail a first-class letter to the
author c/o Inner Traditions • Bear & Company, One Park Street, Rochester, VT
05767, and we will forward the communication.

CONTENTS

A NOTE TO THE READER
Before Beginning the Book

This book is intended to help men who are experiencing low androgen levels and the attendant physical and emotional problems that go along with them. It is also intended to introduce to a wider audience the idea of phytoandrogens, that is, plants that contain male hormones. While work on phytoestrogens, plants that contain female hormones, is fairly advanced and widely known, the concept of phytoandrogens is not.

In general, the material in this book is intended for men over 40. Few men under that age need hormone replacement therapy. When men move into their own midlife shift, a shift that is equal in its impacts to the one experienced by women at menopause, the process is often difficult. The difficulty comes from two sources. The first is our culture's lack of recognition of and support for this shift in maleness. The second is the scores to hundreds of chemicals that are present in the environment that act as endocrine disruptors, that is, they affect, often significantly, the hormonal balance in the male body.

The use of plants as foods and medicines can often alleviate many of the problems men experience during the midlife shift. Some of these plants contain testosterone, molecularly identical to that produced in our bodies. Many possess other androgens or androgen analogues; some act through specific mechanisms to keep testosterone levels high.

In each section of the book, in order to facilitate easy access to the information the plant, supplement, and food protocols are usually outlined in a box at the beginning of that chapter. You may use any or all of these protocols to enhance your levels of testosterone. As with all protocols intended to alter physical states, you should pay close attention to your own body and determine just which ones work best for you. You, after all, know yourself better than anyone else ever will. You will know if these things work for you, what dosages are best, and how long you need to take them. What I offer here are guidelines only, the beginning of a dialogue about more natural means to help men through this shift. It is my hope that men will come to explore their own midlife shifting, that wide recognition of the importance and process of that shift occurs, and that each generation of men will eventually be supported in this move into a new kind of maleness.

The information and plants in this book helped me a great deal and it is my hope that they will help you as well.

"Illegitimi non carborundum"

1 THE IMPORTANCE OF NATURAL HORMONE SUPPORT FOR MEN

*All of us have two lives: the life we learn with and the
life we live with after.*

GLENN CLOSE, IN *THE NATURAL*

One of the more amusing stories about scientific research details the year-long, $100,000 program to determine why children fall off their tricycles. After several well-designed studies were completed and the highly degreed researchers had compiled and analyzed their data, they found that children fall off their tricycles because they lose their balance.

This story often comes back to me when I read various pronouncements from members of the medical profession, and never more often than when I read that there is no such thing as andropause (male menopause). Essentially, they say that because no study has found it, it does not exist. The comments of millions of men that they just don't feel like themselves and that something is wrong are passed off as psychological—our minds playing tricks on us. This same kind of denial has also occurred when discussing women's reproductive conditions, such as menstruation, pregnancy, and menopause. In response, women have pioneered research and exploration into the changes that occur for them during these times and none more so than those that occur during their passage into menopause. Men are long overdue for their own exploration into this territory because the changes that we experience are just as profound, just as life altering, and just as pervasive as those experienced by women. Although it is true that men, at advanced ages, can still participate in creating children and women cannot, there are significant alterations in men's hormonal chemistries as they age, just as there are with women.

Sudden shifts in body chemistries occur for all of us during the major passages in human life: birth, adolescence, middle age, old age, and death. Most of us can remember our shift into adolescence. Our bodies were changing radically, preparing us for reproduction and independence. At the same time, just as significantly, our minds and spirits were shifting, preparing us for life as adults, for love and families of our own, for careers, and our individual and unique destinies.

These shifts had tremendous physical and emotional impacts as we moved into adolescence. Our bodies changed shape, our skin altered, we began growing hair in places it had not grown before, and our voices deepened. In short, our entire appearance changed. And, just as significant, how the world saw us changed. We had to get used to a new "image," a new "face." The person we saw when we looked in mirrors, those at home and those in people's eyes, had changed. The young boy we had been was gone, and a new someone had come to take his place. At the same time, a similar process was occurring in our minds and spirits. New options for life were opening up and the world of sex lay before us, with vast horizons of reproductive options and attractive bodies in endless variation. We were learning new interaction styles and figuring out where we wanted to go, what we wanted to do, and who we wanted to be as adults. A certain force of personality, an older self, had begun to take us over and come into being.

That new way of being—the physical, emotional, and spiritual processes of an adolescent and young adult that came into being as we moved out of childhood—had a certain life span, a certain arc, a period of growth, development, maturity, and then senescence or ending. A transition process, in many ways similar to adolescence, occurs again when we enter the middle of life. We look in the mirror and notice that someone new is taking the place of that young man we were. Then, one day, we mildly flirt with a young woman, much as we always have done since our movement into adolescence, and instead of the usual response, one we had become used to over long years of social interaction, the response we get is different. Her eyes respond with, "You're old enough to be my father." In that moment, the changes that have begun catch up with us. We, whether we want to or not, have entered middle age.

Daily, this new truth is reflected back to us. We look in the eyes of attractive women, and the reflection we see is strange, distorted, and middle-aged. A certain shock runs through our system, and we begin to grapple with our own aging process and the end of an earlier, important period of male life. As with adolescence, there are emotional and spiritual components that are essential aspects to this change as well. We begin to examine our lives, to see what we have done and have not done, to sum up, and to take stock. Our function as a man begins to change. Now it is not so much concerned with the reproduction of children but with something else, something that our society is not so clear about, so it is harder to identify, harder to grasp. This cultural unclarity as so many of us find out, makes it harder to resolve this change, this shifting that occurs in mid life. At the same time, we notice our body *is* older. The impacts of twenty or thirty years of riotous, reproductive living, of raising children, learning our trades, surviving our mistakes have all taken their toll. Parts of our bodies are not working as well as they once did. As with adolescence, our bodies are ready for something else, some other function, a function that our society is not so clear about. And so we struggle with that during this midlife change.

The United States is a young country. In many ways our culture is still an adolescent and, as such, is concerned with adolescent things: sex and reproduction, protection of territory, making money, asserting independence, the freedom to do and say what we want, and being top dog. All these things are integral to the movement into adolescence and young adulthood. However, in middle age something else begins to happen. Because our culture is so unclear about what that is, each of us struggles perhaps more than we should with what we are becoming and the new tasks that lie before us. Many of us begin to realize that although it is true that if you are not top dog the view never changes, if you are top dog, the dogs behind you always see you as one thing. We begin to see that there is something other than the adolescent drives that we have known for so long.

Historically, many cultures have understood this transition much better than we now do. Middle age was recognized for its importance, as were the tasks that lay before the newly awakening middle-aged man. The Jungian analyst James Hillman is one of the few writers struggling to understand the territory of middle and old age and its importance. In his book *The Force of Character and the Lasting Life,* he makes a deeply insightful point when he remarks:

> The transition [to middle age] is first of all psychological, and to me it means this: It is not we who are leaving, but a set of attitudes and interpretations regarding the body and the mind that have outlasted their usefulness—and their youthfulness. We are being forced to leave them behind. They can no longer sustain us, not because we are old, but because *they* are old.[1]

Middle age and old age are not simply the wearing out of the body but also the movement into new territories of self, into new tasks as human beings. As Hillman goes on to say, "Aging is no accident. It is necessary to the human condition, intended by the soul." Emotionally, we are, in fact, coming to terms with our youth, thinking it over. The dreams of who we would become, made during adolescence, are pulled out of the cupboard, dusted off, and examined. We compare them to what we have actually done. Then we look over who we are and what we want to do now. It is common to be less interested in the accumulation of power, reproduction, or making money and more interested in the respect of our peers, intimacy, and developing a new wealth of experience of the world. Often, men become more interested in learning, travel, and helping younger generations through their own struggles with young adulthood. We see our children into adulthood and our parents out. We look at who we are and discover important things that we must still accomplish, and often we leave one career and begin another, one more concerned, quite often, with deeper aesthetic values.

After this transition, men remain vital, strong, and possessed of new insights, tasks, skills, and strengths. Yet we *are* different. A new form of man has emerged. There is, in fact, a unique ego state that emerges, one as distinctive as that of the two-year-old, the four-year-old, or the adolescent. Like those other crucial developmental ego states, this one, too, is biologically encoded to emerge at a specific time, for a specific reason.

The lack of understanding in our culture of the importance of this new developmental stage of the self, of what it means, what it is for, and just how to move into it gracefully, makes the transition all the more difficult. We enter new territories of self that must be encountered, explored, and experimented with in order for them to be fully realized and for this new way of being to be integrated and whole. Of necessity, we must grieve the loss of that older self, the young man with whom we have lived so long. Eventually, if the territory is fully entered and fully encountered, its shape, its terrain, begins to make sense. We begin to find out who we are now and what we are meant to do. There is a celebration of sorts, and many of us come to know ourselves and our purposes here better than we ever have.

All of this takes work. It takes time, and if we are lucky, we can take that time away from work and family and the responsibilities that we have undertaken over the years of our lives. We can take the time to journey inside ourselves and to do this work in interior time.

This would be challenging enough were it the only thing to be dealt with, but there is another factor that makes it harder still, a factor that interferes with the successful transition into a healthy, vital middle age: the pervasiveness of chemicals throughout the ecosystem that mimic the actions of estrogens (female hormones). The powerful and historically unique presence of these chemistries in our ecosystem and on our bodies cannot be overstated. Their daily intake, through our food and water, alters the hormonal balance of our bodies and, during the shift into middle age, exacerbates the normal changes that our bodies are biologically intended to make. This results, quite often, not only in loss of energy and libido, but in a number of disease conditions that commonly plague men in later life: infertility, impotence, heart disease, and so on.

During our shift into middle age, our body chemistry begins to change. Testosterone and other androgen (male hormone) levels start to shift in important ways. Our bodies broaden out, our ears grow bigger and longer, hair, once again, begins to appear in unusual places (and disappear in others). These are normal changes. They and many others are elements of our shift into another kind of maleness. But something is interfering with this natural shift of our bodies. Researchers who study the endocrine system now realize that environmental estrogenic pollutants and substances are entering our bodies in tremendous quantities. When they do so, they shift the balance from testosterone (and other androgens) toward the estrogen side of the equation. Like women, we do have estrogens in our bodies (just as they have testosterone), we just don't have the same quantities, and we have a great deal more testosterone than they do. What is most important is the ratio of androgens to estrogens. Anything that upsets that balance changes who and what we become. We are not our chemistry, but we certainly are affected by our chemistry. The power of our androgenic chemistry to shape who we are begins while we are still in the womb.

2 ANDROPAUSE
Hormones and the Male Body

Although men are accused of not knowing their
own weaknesses, yet perhaps as few know their own
strength. It is in men as in soils, where sometimes there
is a vein of gold which the owner knows not of.

JONATHAN SWIFT

There are essentially four kinds of hormones in our bodies, and they are typed depending on what kind of molecule they are built from. Sexual hormones such as testosterone are built around a specific type of molecule, a sterol, from which the word *steroid* comes. You are familiar with the name of the particular sterol that is used for sexual hormones—cholesterol. It is, in fact, cholesterol from which all steroid hormones are made.

Adrenaline is another kind of hormone that serves as a source of energy during the flight-or-fight response. It is built around an amino acid called tyrosine (as is the thyroid hormone thyroxine) in the adrenal gland. Another type of hormone, insulin, which is highly important in the body's ability to utilize glucose (a kind of sugar) effectively, is built in the pancreas using complex proteins. Others are built around short-chain amino acids called peptides.

Hormones regulate much of the functioning of our bodies. Through complex biofeedback loops, our bodies determine exactly what their needs are at any one moment in time and either make or release hormones to shift their functioning in the direction it needs to go. As an example of this kind of generalized biofeedback, there is no central thermostat in our bodies that keeps them at a certain temperature. Despite the famous 98.6° redlined on so many thermometers, the temperature of the body shifts constantly; it is always in flux. The various systems of the body compare notes as it were and together, in some manner not understood by scientists, come to a conclusion about how temperature needs to shift and then shift it. We are more a collection of cooperating parts, each with its own innate intelligence, than a mechanical system with the brain acting as intelligent overseer. Our hormone levels are, as well, constantly in flux. Our bodies make and release hormones as we need them to remain vital and healthy. Part of this process includes the making and releasing of sexual hormones. In middle age, the amount of testosterone in male bodies naturally shifts, as does the balance between androgens and estrogens. It is the movement toward excess levels of estrogen and the overreduction of testosterone that produces a great many of the problems that men face as they age.

THE SEXUAL HORMONES

Women's sexual hormones are collectively known as estrogens, the main ones being estradiol, estrone, estriol, and 16a-hydroxyestrone. Estradiol is the most pervasive and the strongest in its effects, much like testosterone in males. Progesterone, not usually considered an estrogen, is another female steroid hormone that most people have heard of.

Men's sexual hormones are collectively known as androgens, the primary ones being testosterone, androstenedione (andro), androstenediol, dihydrotestosterone (DHT), dehydroepiandrosterone (DHEA), and dehydroepiandrosterone sulfate (DHEAS), a slightly more complex form of DHEA.

The precursor to all these hormones is cholesterol, which is converted, in sequence, into the steroid hormones pregnenolone and 17a-hydroxypregnenolone. Essentially, pregnenolone is the primary steroid hormone that is converted, or metabolized, into all the other steroid hormones in both women and men; for this reason, it is sometimes referred to as a prohormone. Other people sometimes refer to it as the "mother" steroid, which I guess would make cholesterol the "grandmother." All women have some androgens, all men have some estrogens. Each is important in the healthy functioning of our bodies.

In women, estrogens are made in the ovaries, adrenal glands (which sit on top of the kidneys), and brain. Increasingly, research is revealing that both androgens and estrogens also act as potent neurohormones that strongly affect central nervous system activity, which is why both estrogens and androgens are produced in the brain and central nervous system.

Androgens are made in men's testicles, adrenal glands, brain, and peripheral tissues and cells—that is, any muscle tissue or any other cell or organ in the body that needs androgens for a particular function at a specific time. About 95 percent of testosterone is made in a man's testes, most of the rest is made in the adrenal glands, and a small amount is made in peripheral tissues and cells. Other androgens (such as DHEA and DHEAS) are made in the brain from precursors or prohormones like pregnenolone. The two sexual hormones that seem to be the most important, at least on the surface, are estradiol in women and testosterone in men.

Everyone knows that testosterone makes a man a man. Its presence in our bodies literally does make us men. Testosterone peaks three times in our lives. During the second trimester of fetal development, blood levels of testosterone increase from nearly zero to about 4.0 nanograms per milliliter (ng/mL). (A nanogram is a billionth of a gram, and a milliliter is 0.034 of an ounce.) This is a tremendously tiny amount, yet it causes the fetus to develop as male. Then after birth, testosterone begins to rise again, peaks around six months of age at about 2.5 ng/mL, and drops slowly back to near zero by age one. Part of the purpose of this surge in testosterone after birth is to initiate the formation of the prostate gland. Still, the gland remains tiny, weighing only one to two grams. The final rise in testosterone begins between ages ten and eleven and rises slowly to a peak of about 5.0 ng/mL around the age of eighteen. Then it holds relatively steady until sometime around the age of forty-five, when it very slowly declines throughout the rest of life. During this last rise of testosterone in adolescence, the penis, scrotum, and prostate gland all enlarge, the voice deepens, facial and body hair begins to grow, sperm production begins, the bones lengthen and grow more massive, and the body expands rapidly to a much larger size.

Because the overall testosterone levels in the body that physicians usually test for (as opposed to free testosterone, which is something I will talk about later) remain roughly the same after age forty-five, because men can still father children after that age, and because there is not a sudden, comparable, shift in body functions similar to that which women experience during the cessation of menstruation, many physicians and researchers have insisted that there is no such thing as a male menopause and that, in spite of so many men experiencing it, it is all in our heads. Other researchers, who do not accept this perspective, however, have found two interesting things. The first is that while the overall levels of total testosterone remain relatively constant, *free* testosterone levels do change considerably. The second is that the androgen/estrogen ratio shifts significantly as well.

Of the testosterone in the male body, 70 to 80 percent is bound to a protein—sex hormone binding globulin (SHBG). Another 20 percent or so is bound to a different protein—albumin. Bound testosterone is used up, not available, doing something else. Only free testosterone, which makes up 1 to 3 percent of the body's total testosterone level, is completely biologically available and active at the receptor sites of testosterone target cells. As we age, the amounts of these testosterone types alter considerably, which contributes to the alterations men experience in middle age. SHBG bound testosterone increases nearly 80 percent by age ninety. By age 100, free testosterone will usually disappear entirely. The Massachusetts Male Aging Study, conducted at the New England Research Institute in Watertown, MA, found that, in general, in healthy men the amount of free testosterone declines an average of 1.2 percent per year between the ages of thirty-nine and seventy.[1] During this same period, albumin-bound testosterone declines around 1.0 percent per year, while SHBG-bound testosterone and body levels of SHBG increase 1.2 percent per year. But, bound testosterone is only part of the story. During the same time period, the quantity of testosterone that is converted to other substances increases as well.

Testosterone itself is not an end product. It gets converted into other substances that the body needs. For instance, an enzyme called aromatase converts testosterone to the estrogen estradiol, and another enzyme, 5-alpha reductase, converts testosterone to DHT, which many people consider the most potent androgenic substance of all (and the actual hormone that does what testosterone has long been thought to do). DHT is a potent androgen, while estradiol is a potent estrogen. In many respects, estradiol can be considered the substance that makes women women. So, the substance that testosterone is converted into (DHT or estradiol) has tremendous impacts on male health and well-being.

In small amounts, estradiol in men is crucial in supporting the health and growth of the neural filaments in the brain, which connect brain cells to each other. Estradiol is also crucial in the creation and maintenance of the essential brain neurotransmitter acetylcholine. Estradiol and other estrogens in the male body also support healthy sexual functioning, blood and arterial flow, skin health, and so on. During the middle-age shift, male bodies naturally begin to have a bit more estradiol than they did when younger. This contributes to some of the changes we experience. But, if too much testosterone is converted to estradiol, the androgen/estrogen balance is significantly altered and this can have tremendous impacts on how we feel as men. It can affect our levels of health as well.

The increasing loss of free testosterone over time creates significant alterations in our bodies and our experiences of ourselves. (Remember, we are male simply from exposure to tiny nanogram quantities of testosterone while we were in the womb.) And, at the same time, we are experiencing *more* estrogenic hormones which, at the same tiny nanogram levels, make women who they are. It is no wonder that so many men's experience of themselves and their lives change so much as they begin entering their forties and fifties.

It is this shift in free testosterone levels and the changing androgen/estrogen ratio together that signals our movement into middle age. Hormonal shifting as we move into new stages of life is something that our bodies naturally do, much as when as infants in the womb we released the chemicals that began our mother's contractions leading to our birth. These hormonal shifts occur at different ages for every man and no one can predict why, how, or when they will naturally occur. It is an expression of our unique selves: genetic history, body chemistry, environment, beliefs, stresses, foods, hopes, dreams, aspirations, losses, grievings, loves, and destiny. It is a natural occurrence, not an inevitable *decline*, not a disease. It simply is a shift into a new way of being, a new expression of maleness.

Unfortunately, this is where environmental pollutants become a problem. Industrial substances in the millions of tons are entering the environment each year and having tremendous impacts on male sexual health. They are exacerbating the movement into middle age that men naturally experience. Researchers have found that some of these substances cause more testosterone to be converted to estradiol, others actually interfere with the production of testosterone, and still others are potent estrogens that, as they are taken into our bodies, seriously disrupt the androgen/estrogen balance. For many of us, androgen levels are so profoundly affected that sexual vitality and quality of life are significantly reduced.

3 ENVIRONMENTAL POLLUTANT IMPACTS ON TESTOSTERONE

It is not a debate about whether [endocrine disruption] is happening or not. It is happening. We just have to decide to what degree we want to let it continue to happen.

LOUIS GUILLETTE

There is significant evidence that scores of substances, usually synthetic chemicals that either are estrogens or mimic estrogens, are entering men's bodies and significantly altering the androgen/estrogen ratio far beyond the normal range that men have historically experienced. Some of these environmental pollutants also have the capacity to bind free testosterone and to interfere with its creation or its proper levels in our bodies. This is affecting younger males, often through estrogenic impacts in the womb prior to their birth, as well as older men. Some of the impacts are extremely sobering. As a result of these external (or exogenous) estrogens, Peter Montague of *Rachel's Environment and Health Weekly* (now *Rachel's Democracy and Health News*) observed:

> Each year more men in the industrialized world are getting cancer of the testicles [and prostate], birth defects affecting the penis, lowered sperm count, lowered sperm quality, and undescended testicles.[1]

The degree of this shift in male androgen levels is a relatively new occurrence. It began in a very mild way in Europe in 1516 with the passage of the German Beer Purity Act (see the section on hops in chapter 7), spread very slowly for three hundred years, and then began escalating with the discovery and production of synthetic chemicals in industry. Researchers have found that the shifts in male androgen levels and ratios we are now seeing come from hundreds of synthetically produced estrogenic chemicals (estrogen mimics) as well as androgen antagonists or antiandrogens that directly deactivate androgens in our bodies. The past sixty years have seen an evolutionarily unprecedented proliferation of these kinds of synthetic chemicals. One-third of American men, about thirty million of us, are estimated to be experiencing some form of erectile dysfunction or impotence. But, the males of every species, not just humans, are paying the price of these estrogenic pollutants.

THE EFFECTS OF ESTROGEN MIMICS AND ANDROGEN ANTAGONISTS ON MALE HEALTH

Over the past fifty years, scientists have recorded a frightening shift in men's reproductive health. Sperm counts are showing a significant decline worldwide, testicular cancer has grown at approximately 2 to 4 percent per year in men under fifty years of age, a general increase in cryptorchidism (undescended testes) has occurred in young men, and general increases in hypospadia (penile deformities) have been seen.[2] The increases in testicular cancer, for instance, parallel almost exactly the historical rise in production of synthetic chemicals—industrial, agrochemical, and pharmaceutical. From 1880 to 1920, there was virtually no change in testicular cancer rates. After 1920, they began to rise steadily in direct proportion to the amount of synthetic chemicals that were being produced worldwide.[3]

Estrogenic Pollution

These kinds of reproductive problems are being seen in the males of scores of species throughout the world: panthers, birds, fish, alligators, frogs, bats, turtles, and many more. Louis Guillette, a reproductive endocrinologist and professor of zoology at the University of Florida, is an expert on the study of endocrine-disrupting chemicals in the environment. He has spent years studying the effects of environmental endocrine disruptors (chemicals that interfere with the activity of sexual hormones). His research on male alligators, he notes, has consistently shown that androgen levels, androgen ratios, and free testosterone levels are all significantly altered by environmental pollutants and have been for some time. "In males," Guillette writes, "this abnormality in testosterone persists, so there is a dramatic change in circulating levels of testosterone. DHT is altered as well, and some males have elevated levels of estrogens. So there are feminized males."[4] He comments that the levels of chemicals needed to produce such changes are incredibly tiny. "We did not [test] one part per trillion for the contaminant, as we assumed that was too low. Well, we were wrong. It ends up that everything from a hundred parts per trillion to ten parts per million are ecologically relevant . . . at these levels there is sex reversal . . . [And our research] shows that the highest dose does not always give the greatest response. That has been a very disturbing issue for many people trying to do risk assessment in toxicology."[5]

Pharmaceutical-quality steroids are in fact extremely pervasive in world ecosystems. They are entering soil, air, and water in the millions of tons from farming and the heavy use of estrogenic pharmaceuticals by women worldwide. Birth control pills and menopausal hormone replacement therapies are especially pervasive sources of estrogenic pollution. The synthetic estrogen Premarin, for example, is the most widely prescribed pharmaceutical in the United States. Pharmaceuticals such as these are excreted out of the human body and enter the environment, where they continue to be active as steroidal chemicals. Researchers commonly find synthetic estradiol, the most potent estrogen, and another estrogen, estrone, in wastewater coming from sewage plants. They have regularly found concentrations of estradiol at 14 parts per trillion (ppt) and estrone at 400 ppt. All of the male fish downstream from such concentrations of estrogen pollution have been found to exhibit sexual reproductive problems, many of them becoming female. Researchers testing the potency of these estrogens found that sex changes begin at the incredibly tiny levels of 0.1 ppt of estradiol and 10 ppt of estrone.[6]

DDT and Other Chemicals

Other chemicals such as dichlorodiphenyltrichloroethane (DDT), organo-chlorines, polychlorinated biphenyls (PCBs), and their metabolites (the chemicals they are metabolized into) are strongly active as estrogen mimics and are prevalent throughout the world's soils, water, and air. Millions of tons of these estrogen mimics are used as pesticides on farms throughout the world. Especially impactful are huge agribusiness operations, which use these kinds of chemicals in tremendous quantities to increase animal growth.

Although people in the United States think that DDT is ancient history, it is not. Although it is not used in the United States, it is still common in other parts of the world. In fact, in 1995 more DDT was used than at any previous time in history.[7] The United States is not an ecologically isolated country, and chemicals such as DDT circulate in the atmosphere and oceans, so there are still measurable amounts of DDT throughout the soil and water of the United States. DDT is, in fact, a globally pervasive chemical. Recent studies have regularly found DDT in the blood of North American wildlife at average concentrations of 1 nanogram per milliliter. This is about 1,000 times higher than the normal blood levels of free estradiol (which DDT mimics) that should be found in wildlife.[8] And p,p'-DDE, a breakdown byproduct of DDT, has been found to be a powerful androgen antagonist, strongly interfering with male androgen balances and levels in all male species that encounter it.[9] The common pesticide vinclozolin, used on agricultural products such as cucumbers, grapes, lettuce, onions, bell peppers, raspberries, strawberries, and tomatoes, is also a powerful androgen antagonist. Sold under the trade names Ronilan, Ornalin, Curalan, and Voralan and mixed as a part of products such as Hitrun, Kinker, Ronilan M, Ronilan T Combi, Silbos, and Fungo-50, it is widely available for agricultural and gardening use. One of its breakdown byproducts (a metabolite) has been found to be 100 times more powerful than vinclozolin as an androgen antagonist.[10] Some of the environmental pollutants, such as the fungicide propiconazole, are so strong that numerous researchers have begun exploring the use of their active chemicals (imidazole derivatives) as male contraceptives.[11] Pyrimidine carbinol fungicides are so potent that they can actually inhibit all hormone production. They completely block the synthesis of sterols, including cholesterol, from which all steroid hormones are made.[12]

Phthalates, used widely in medicine to make plastics flexible, have also been found to significantly affect androgen-dependent tissues.[13] Health Care Without Harm, an organization trying to help minimize the negative health impacts from hospitals and medical technology, notes that although some phthalates act as estrogen mimics, others are powerful androgen antagonists. One phthalate, DEHP (Di-[2-ethylhexyl] phthalate), and its metabolite, MEHP (mono-[2-ethylhexyl] phthalate), show significant testicular toxicity, especially to the testes' Sertoli cells. The Sertoli cells nurse immature sperm to maturity, and phtalate-related chemical toxicity results in decreased sperm production. Simply using medical devices (such as plasma bags or tubing) that contain DEHP can result in significant drops in sperm health because the phthalates readily leach out of the plastic and into the human body.[14] Dioxins and plastics that contain polyvinyl chloride (PVC) produce similar kinds of impacts on male health.

Concerns of Environmental Groups

The environmental group Greenpeace has raised concern about just a few of the synthetic chemicals that are known to be hormone disruptors, including the following:

- Eleven common pesticides and their metabolites
- PCBs (still environmentally present although no longer produced)
- Dioxins and furans (by-products of chlorine production and the chlorinated plastic PVC)
- Bisphenol A (an ingredient used in dental fillings and to coat the inside of tin cans and reusable milk bottles)

- Phthalates (used to make plastic flexible in such things as checkbook covers, medical tubing, baby teething rings)
- Butylated hydroxyanisole (BHA) a food additive[15]

Increasingly, these substances are being found to have direct impacts on male reproductive health. As the authors of *Our Stolen Future* report, "Several studies report that infertile men have higher levels of PCBs and other synthetic chemicals in their blood or semen, and one analysis found a correlation between the swimming ability of a man's sperm and the concentration of [PCBs] found in his semen."[16]

It is not only environmental groups that are concerned. Scientific organizations and environmental agencies in countries throughout the world have come to the inescapable conclusion that male health in every species on Earth is being negatively affected by these synthetic chemicals.

As only one example, the Danish Environmental Protection Agency released a report in 1995 titled "Male Reproductive Health and Environmental Chemicals with Estrogenic Effects." The 175-page report identified numerous consumer products that contain known hormone-disrupting chemicals such as "pesticides, detergents, cosmetics, paints, and packaging materials including plastic containers and food wraps."[17] Ten classes of chemicals containing hundreds of different types of products were listed as agents of concern.

Peter Montague reflects that the report makes clear that "in contrast [to natural hormones], many industrial chemicals that enter the body are not readily broken down so they circulate in the blood for long periods—in some cases many years—mimicking natural hormones."[18] What is worse, these hormonally active substances can combine with each other in ways that are not understood, are not predictable, and have never been studied.

Effects of Pollutants

The impacts of these kinds of chemicals on our lives and our movements through the stages of our lives as men cannot be overstated. It is tremendously important to recognize that many of the contemporary difficulties that men are experiencing in middle age or even as young adults are the result of the pervasive intake of nanogram-sized quantities of these chemicals. Prostate problems, erectile dysfunction, sterility, sperm motility problems, loss of energy, libido, and even atherosclerosis (fat-clogged arteries), heart disease, and many more common physical problems can be tied to the disruption of the androgen/estrogen balance and the dropping levels of free testosterone in our bodies. In 1920, men in the United States had the same life expectancy as women. As increasing numbers of estrogenic-like substances entered the environment and our bodies, our life expectancy has dropped until we now lag eight years behind women.

The pervasive problem of these chemicals is being compounded by the significant shift in the foods we eat. Over the million years of our evolutionary history, human beings lived as a part of their forest and savanna homes. Normally, they ate several hundred to several thousand kinds of plants each year as a regular part of their diet. Our human bodies have been used to that kind of food intake for a million years; they expect it and need it. The majority of these plants are filled with hundreds to thousands of potent natural chemicals that we need to remain healthy. On average, people in the industrialized nations now eat from five to twelve vegetables per year. Most of the vegetables have been modified for taste, which has reduced or eliminated many of their most potent chemical components.

The combination of these converging historical events is ensuring that men do not enter middle age in vital health as we historically have done. This is why it becomes important for many of us to actively work in some fashion to restore our natural levels and ratios of androgens.

4 PHYTOANDROGENS
Natural Hormone Replacement Therapy for Men

As they fell from heaven, the plants said, "whichever
living soul we pervade, that man will suffer no harm."
THE RIG-VEDA

While it is true that for many of us our hormonal balance has been disturbed and our levels of free testosterone have been falling, it is possible to reverse this process by regularly supplementing the diet with plants high in androgens, natural steroidal supplements and vitamins, and androgen-stimulating foods. Incorporating these as a regular part of your diet for from two weeks to one year can enhance free testosterone levels and positively alter the androgen/estrogen ratio. The rest of this book will look at the most important plants, supplements, and foods that can be used to increase testosterone levels and alter the androgen/ estrogen balance toward the androgen side of the equation. This chapter will look at a unique class of plant medicines—phytoandrogens.

PHYTOANDROGENS AND HEALTH IN MIDDLE-AGED MEN

The concept of phytoandrogens, meaning plants that contain androgens or those that stimulate androgenic activity in men, is relatively new. Phytoestrogens have a much deeper history, and most clinicians and many people have at least some idea of their existence. Phytoandrogens do the same things that phytoestrogens do, except they do it for men and they do not supply estrogens, they provide androgens. Phytoandrogens increase the body's levels of free testosterone, and they shift the androgen/estrogen balance more toward the androgen side of the equation.

Plants do this by directly supplying androgens such as testosterone, stimulating the body's production of androgens, or by interfering with the breakdown (or conversion) of androgens into estrogens or their binding to SHBG (see chapter 2) or albumin. Pine pollen is an example of a plant that supplies significant quantities of testosterone and other androgens. The ginsengs (asian, tienchi, eleutherococcus) and tribulus are examples of plants that stimulate the production of androgens in the body. Nettle root is an example of a plant that prevents the conversion of testosterone into estrogens and interferes with its binding to inert substances in the body.

Plants that contain testosterone are ubiquitous in the environment, but very little research has been done on them. Hopefully, as knowledge of phytoandrogens becomes more widespread, research will follow along. There are a great many plants out there that contain testosterone or other androgens; it's just that no one has been looking for them.

The following herbs are some of the most powerful phytoandrogens known so far. The plant that contains the most testosterone (and other androgens) is, at this point, pine, especially its pollen. Over the past ten years, I have experienced a great deal of benefit from it, as have a great many men from whom I have heard. David's lily also contains substantial amounts, but at this time it is not commercially available. My own experience is that it is not as strong as pine pollen, perhaps because it must be harvested within a tiny window of time when it reaches peak testosterone production, something that is not always possible. It is included here in the hope that the information on it will stimulate commercial growers to make it available. All the other herbs are easy to find. Sources for all herbs, except David's lily, are listed in the resource section at the end of the book.

The combination protocol outlined here will reliably act to increase testosterone levels, general energy levels, and overall sense of well-being.

Natural Testosterone Enhancement Protocol

Pine pollen tincture: ⅜ tsp. three times per day

Nettle root: 1200 mg per day

Tribulus: 500 mg three times per day

Panax ginseng: ¼ tsp. daily

Tienchi ginseng: ⅓ tsp. three times per day

Eleuthero: 1 tsp. twice a day

Pine (*Pinus spp.*) and Pine Pollen (*Pollen pini*)

Family: Pinaceae

Common Names: Pine. Specific species have different names: Scots or Scotch pine *(Pinus sylvestris)*, black pine *(Pinus nigra)*, Korean pine *(Pinus koraiensis)*, masson pine *(Pinus massonia)*, Chinese pine, aka Chinese oil pine, aka Chinese red pine *(Pinus tabulaeformis)*.

Primary Species Used: Although all pine pollens contain testosterone, the primary species of trees used for their pollen are *P. sylvestris* and *P. nigra* in the United States, *P. koraiensis* in Korea, and *P. massonia* and *P. tabulaeformis* in China. Any species, however, will do.

Parts Used: All parts of the pine are used for medicine: the pollen, bark, seeds, and needles. To increase testosterone in the body and balance the androgen/estrogen ratio, the pollen is the primary part used. It is very high in testosterone. To a lesser extent, the seeds may also be used for this purpose, with some caveats (see chapter 6). Although the bark is excellent for many things, it normally does not contain enough testosterone and other androgens to be of use for this purpose.

Common Names for Pine Pollen: English: pine pollen, Chinese: Songhuanfen, Korean: songhwaju, Latin: pollen pini. **NOTE:** a number of sources and Web sites translate *pollen pini* as "bee pollen" and sell bee pollen as pollen pini—this is incorrect. When looking for pine pollen, care must be taken that what they are labeling pollen pini really is pine pollen and not bee pollen.

Habitat: Worldwide, there are some 100 species of pines. In general, they are native to the temperate and mountainous regions of the Northern Hemisphere. They range from the arctic as far south as North Africa, the Philippines, and Central America. Only one species is indigenous south of the equator, *Pinus merkusii,* which is native to Sumatra. However, many pine species have experienced human distribution south of the equator and now grow wild wherever they were introduced. Of the species used for pine pollen, *P. sylvestris,* for example, is native to Europe from Norway to Spain and parts of Asia. It prefers a well-drained, acidic soil with full sun. It is very tolerant of dry, infertile soils.

Cultivation: Pines, especially *Pinus sylvestris,* easily cultivate from seeds.

Collection: The season for collecting pine pollen usually occurs from March to May in the northern latitudes. Mid-April is often a prime collecting period.

The male catkins that grow in a clump at the end of pine branches each look somewhat like a small, curved, corn-on-the-cob or perhaps small, curved cattails. These catkins produce the pollen that sometimes covers the ground with blankets of yellow powder during the pollen season. The catkins are collected when the pollen production is highest. In China, the catkins are placed in open tray containers to dry. Then the catkins are shaken, the pollen separated, and the catkins discarded. Because digestibility by humans of raw pine pollen is (according to producers) limited, the Chinese producers of pine pollen tablets and powders crush the pollen grains to break the cell walls before they are sold.

In the United States, the main producer of pine pollen tincture collects the pollen-laden catkins during peak pollen season and tinctures them. That is, they are placed, fresh, in a water and alcohol mix to macerate. The tincture, at maturity, is strained and stored in amber bottles out of direct sunlight.

Actions of Pine Pollen: Strongly androgenic, increases free testosterone levels in blood, restores androgen/estrogen balance, highly nutritive (strong amino acid and vitamin source), stimulates liver regeneration, reduces blood cholesterol levels, increases superoxide dismutase levels (SOD; a potent antioxidant) in heart, liver and brain, enhances immunity, and supports healthy endocrine function.

Actions of Pine Seeds: Moderately androgenic, strongly nutritive.

Actions of Pine Bark: Mildly androgenic, potent antioxidant, free-radical scavenger, and lipid peroxidation inhibitor, anti-inflammatory, collagen and elastin stabilizer.

Chemistry: Pine pollen contains large quantities of sterols, steroid-like substances, that are exceptionally potent. Many of these are brassinosteroids. One such, brassinoloide, is a powerful growth stimulant to plants. As little as one nanogram applied to a bean sprout can cause tremendous growth in response. Other brassinosteroids, such as castasterone and typhasterol, are also common in pine pollen. The pollen also contains a variety of endogenous gibberellins and a number of glutathione transferases. Endogenous gibberellins are plant hormones that affect cell enlargement and division. Glutathione transferases possess wide actions in living systems. They detoxify xenobiotics such as chemical carcinogens and environmental pollutants and inactivate unsaturated aldehydes, quinones, and hydroperoxides that occur as metabolites of oxidative stress. More importantly, for this book, they are intimately involved in the biosynthesis of testosterone and progesterone. Plants that grow around pine forests have come to depend on this potent nutrient source for their growth. In fact, brassinosteroids regulate gene expression in many plants. The pollen that falls to the ground or into water is generally taken up very quickly as a food and nutrient growth stimulant by other plants and living organisms in the area, including insects and animals. The brassinosteroids in pollen are actually very similar in structure to many animal steroid hormones and do exhibit steroidal activity. In addition, pine pollen contains significant amounts of human male hormones such as testosterone and androstenedione and relatively large quantities of amino acids, vitamins, minerals, and other nutrients. A more comprehensive look at the components of pine pollen is included under the Scientific Research heading later in this section.

About Pine and Pine Pollen: Pine trees have a long history of use as medicines and foods. Few people now realize that the inner bark of some pines can be harvested in strips and cooked like pasta or that if dried and ground it makes a good flour.

The most androgenic part of pine trees is the pollen, although the seeds and, to a lesser extent, the bark also contain androgens. Seeds may help raise androgen levels in humans when used as a regular food additive, and an extract of the pine's inner bark can be used as a potent antioxidant.

Emerging research has shown that, under certain circumstances, pine bark and the pulp of the tree can be powerfully androgenic. Studies have shown that female fish downstream from pine pulp mills literally transform into males from the high levels of androgens in the water. Analysis of the effluent shows "testosterone-like" impacts, according to researchers. (No other tree effluent produces this result.) The pine species normally used in pine bark extracts is *Pinus pinaster*, which grows along the Atlantic coast of France and into North Africa.

Pine pollen is a yellow, flour-like substance produced in the millions of tons each year by the pine forests of the Earth. Unlike the majority of flowering plants, pine trees are wind-pollinated. That is, they don't have an animal or insect pollinator to help them reproduce but rely on the wind to carry the pollen to the pinecone (the female part of the plant). Each spring, the trees release the pollen from their male catkins, each of which can produce six million grains of pollen. Under magnification, a pollen grain looks much like Mickey Mouse—a big head with two huge cupped ears. The wind catches in the cupped ears, the head acting as a sort of keel hanging underneath, and the pollen sails much like a ship through the air until it finds its way inside the overlapping scale of a cone. The needles around the cones and the cones themselves literally alter wind flow patterns to more accurately funnel the pollen into place so that fertilization can take place. Under each little overlapping scale of a cone, a pine seed, or pine nut, will grow. To facilitate pollination, a great deal more pine pollen is released than is needed, and each spring the ground, streams, and ponds around and under pine forests are covered with the fine yellow pollen powder.

Ayurvedic Use: Pine pollen is unknown in Ayurvedic practice as far as I can determine. A number of pines were used as medicine but mostly the trees, sap, and so on, as antibacterials and for lung complaints. However, the seeds of *P. gerardiana* have a long history of use in India as a tonic aphrodisiac and are considered to be anodyne, stimulants, and nutritive. They were sometimes used for rheumatic complaints, seminal debility, and leukorrhoea and gleet (vaginal and urethral discharges).

Traditional Chinese Medicine: Known as songhuanfen (or song huan fen), pollen from the masson pine, *P. massoniana*, and the Chinese pine, *P. tabulaeformis* (usually blended together) has been used in traditional Chinese medicine for millennia as a health restorative, longevity tonic, and antiaging nutrient. The oldest mention of it in ancient Chinese texts is in *The Pandects of Materia Medica* by Shen Nong of the Han Dynasty (206 BCE–220 CE). Although the herb has been used for several thousand years, current Chinese production methods emphasize breaking the cell wall of the pollen to facilitate absorption. There is little literature I have been able to find that supports the need of this, especially considering the pollen's place in traditional Chinese medicine over such a long period. A low-temperature, high-speed airflow pulverization process is used that breaks up 99 percent of the cellular material.

Traditional Chinese physicians prescribe pine pollen for moistening the lungs, relieving rheumatic pain, relieving fatigue, increasing endurance, strengthening the immune system, improving the skin, strengthening the heart, strengthening the GI tract and stomach, for increasing mental agility, for prostate problems, for increasing agility, and decreasing weight. Interestingly, many of these actions are consistent with the intake of exogenous testosterone. Pine pollen is also used externally as a poultice to arrest discharges, to stop bleeding, and for skin problems such as eczema, impetigo, acne, and diaper rash.

Korean pine pollen (called songhwaju) from *P. koraiensis* is used in Korea in much the same way that similar pine pollen is used in China, often as a tea and also as an additive in many traditional recipes. Although it is becoming harder to find (it is still used regularly in North Korea), pine pollen has traditionally been available in grocery stores in South Korea and is sold in boxes much like those that contain baking soda in the United States. Historically, it has been included regularly in food as an antiaging and invigorating additive.

Western Botanic Practice: Pine pollen has not been a part of traditional Western botanic medicine. It has only recently entered Western botanic practice with the emergence of interest in phytoandrogens.

Scientific Research: Oddly, given its extensive history in China, research on pine pollen in the West is still in its infancy. What researchers have found, however, bears out the Chinese use of pine as an antiaging and vitality-enhancing medicine for men. Pine pollen is extremely high in androgens and the amino acids that support healthy endocrine function. Analysis of pollen from *P. sylvestris, P. nigra, P. bungeana,* and *P. tabulaeformis* has shown the presence of androgenic constituents, including testosterone.

Pinus nigra, or black pine, pollen contains the following androgens: androstenedione (0.7–0.8 mcg per 10 g, 0.000009% by weight), testosterone (0.7 mcg per 10 g, approximately 0.000009% by weight), dehydroepiandrosterone (DHEA; about 0.1 mcg per 10 g, 0.0000015% by weight), and androsterone (approx. 0.2 mcg per 10 g, 0.0000022% by weight). The testosterone in *Pinus bungeana* pollen runs 11 nanograms per 0.1 grams dry weight, and that in *P. tabulaeformis* runs 27 nanograms per 0.1 gram dry weight.

Although these amounts might seem small, recall that it takes as little as four nanograms (one-thousandth of a microgram) to change our sex to men while we are developing in the womb. That can be represented as 0.004 micrograms. Androgens are very potent chemicals. In comparison with that amount, *P. nigra* pollen contains 0.7 micrograms per 10 grams of pollen. The traditional oral dose of pine pollen in China is 4.5 to 9 grams per day.

Amino acid content is high in all pine pollens. For instance, chemical analysis of *Pinus montana* pollen has found that it contains the following amino acids (amounts shown per 100 grams): arginine (6.4 g), leucine (6.5 g), lysine (5.1 g), methionine (1.5 g), phenylalanine (2.1 g), tryptophane (0.8 g), and tyrosine (1.05 g) plus trace amounts of alanine, amino-butyric acid, aspartic acid, cystine, glutamic acid, glycine, hydroxyproline, isoleucine, proline, serine, threonine, and valine.

The *P. massonia* and *P. tabulaeformis* combination that is often used in Chinese pine pollen tablets contains amino acids that are similar to ones in *P. montana,* including the following (amounts shown per 100 grams): asparagic acid (1098 mg), threonine (492 mg), serine (522 mg), amino glutaric acid (1579 mg), aminoacetic acid (698 mg), alanine (564 mg), isoleucine (539 mg), leucine (846 mg), tyrosine (365 mg), phenylalanine (572 mg), lysine (802 mg), histidine (189 mg), cystine (112 mg), valine (646 mg), merionin (166 mg), arginine (998 mg), proline (884 mg), and tryptophan (149 mg).

Phenylalanine is linked with neurotransmitters in the brain and affects mood and dopamine levels in the brain. Both phenylalanine and tyrosine are L-dopa precursors. L-dopa is metabolized into dopamine in both the heart and brain. Without dopamine, neural communication in the brain would be impossible. L-dopa has also been found to increase sexual interest and activity and facilitate erections in men. It is specific for treating anorgasmia, a woman's inability to have an orgasm. Tyrosine is also the precursor for epinephrine (adrenaline) and norepinephrine. Arginine is a precursor of nitric oxide (an erection stimulant) and possesses wound-healing and immune-enhancing functions (which is why pine pollen is so effective for skin conditions). Arginine boosts the release of growth hormones, improves fertility, and is spermigenic (that is, it increases sperm production) at doses of four grams per day.

Pine pollen has been found to be high in vitamins, too. *P. montana* contains the following vitamins (amounts shown per gram of pollen): riboflavin (5.6 mg), nicotinic acid (79.8 mg), pantothenic acid (7.8 mg), pyridoxine (3.1 mg), biotin (0.62 mg), inositol (9 mg), and folic acid (0.42 mg).

Analysis of pine pollen by Chinese researchers has shown similar results. Study has found that it contains (amounts shown per 100 grams): vitamins B_1 (6070 mcg), B_2 (486 mcg), B_6 (1300 mcg), E (3240 mcg), C (562 mcg), D_3 (22.8 mcg), and A (43.2 mcg), nicotinamide (24000 mcg), folic acid (930 mcg), and B-carotin (26.2 mcg).

The amount of vitamin D in *P. sylvestris* and *P. nigra* runs about 2 micrograms per 10 grams of pollen. Vitamins D_2 and D_3 are present in amounts of between 0.1 and 3 micrograms per 10 grams of pollen. The pollen also contains the hydroxylated metabolites of vitamin D_3, which plays an essential role in the regulation of intestinal calcium and phosphorus absorption, calcium mobilization from bone, and reabsorption of calcium and phosphorus in the kidneys. It also modulates osteoclast differentiation, suppression of parathyroid cell growth and parathyroid hormone gene expression and effects growth and differentiation of keratinocytes in skin. This explains, in part, the traditional effectiveness of pine pollen in Chinese medicine to treat people with intestinal complaints and, again, skin problems.

Chinese pine pollen, like all pine pollens, contains numerous essential elements, including the following (amounts shown in parts per million): potassium (3118.8), sodium (516.8), calcium (481), magnesium (1427.5), phosphorus (3609.1), iron (129.9), manganese (280.7), copper (4.3), zinc (9.8), and selenium (0.1). Pine pollens also contain a number of primary constituents. For instance, *P. ponderosa* contains 11.17 percent fatty substances, 0.23 percent ketose sugar, 1.14 percent glucose, 16.40 percent sucrose, and 1.29 percent starch.

Most of the scientific studies have been carried out in China. Few of the papers from these studies have been translated into English. In vivo studies with mice have found that Chinese pine pollen has a distinctive antifatigue effect, enhances survival times under stress, increases SOD activity in the liver, protects the liver from chemical stressors including alcohol, reduces cholesterol levels, increases high density lipoprotein (HDL) levels while reducing low density lipoprotein (LDL) levels, and protects arterial blood vessels from damage. Other in vivo studies of pine pollen have found that it reduces the build up of lipofuscin in the heart, brain, and liver. Lipofuscin is granules of a brown pigment, considered to be an aging pigment, and is the residue of lysomal digestion. Build up of lipofuscin occurs as animals age, and it interferes with healthy function of the organs in which it congregates. Liver spots, for example, are deposits of lipofuscin in the skin. That pine pollen reduces the buildup of lipofuscin in the heart, brain, and liver does give credence to its long use in China as an antiaging herb.

None of the human studies have yet been published in English. Pine pollen's primary use in Chinese medicine has been as an antiaging medicinal that increases male vitality and potency, mental clarity, strength, skin quality, and agility.

Suggested Dosage: Tincture: One full dropper (30 drops, 1.5 mL, or ⅜ tsp.) three times daily or as desired. The tincture is available through www.woodlandessence.com. Tablets: three to six 0.5-gram tablets three times daily (that is, 4.5 to 9 grams daily). See Resources and Sources of Supply section for sources.

Impacts/Importance of Tincture: I have used pine pollen tincture since 2002 and found it extremely effective in practice. When taken as a tincture, the pollen constituents enter the bloodstream almost immediately. There is an immediate upsurge in energy and, over time, an increase in strength, vitality, libido, and optimism. Sexual stamina and erectile function both increase. These effects are commonly reported among users. I am unclear as to whether the androgens in pine pollen tablets will actually enter the bloodstream as effectively, due to the problems that sometimes occur from constituents having to go through digestion and pass through stomach and GI tract membranes. The digestive process sometimes significantly interferes with some constituent absorption. For that reason I think that the tablets are excellent as a supplement on a daily basis but for testosterone enhancement the tincture is a better approach.

Side Effects and Contraindications: Although uncommon, a small percentage of people are allergic to pine pollen. This runs from 1.5 to 10 percent of the population depending on the geographic location. Allergies are usually mild, running from rhinoconjunctivitis (inflammation of the nose and area around the eyeball) to mild asthma in extremely susceptible people. There is one case of anaphylaxis (a severe allergic reaction) to pine nuts in the literature, but such severe effects have not been reported in people using pollen. If you have shown previous sensitivity to pollens, it makes sense to go slow with pine pollen, beginning with a tiny dose, until you are sure that you are not sensitive. **If you have a history of allergies to pollen or severe reactions to bee stings, you should proceed with caution to make sure that your reactions do not extend to pine products.**

Extensive in vivo toxicological tests in China have shown that pine pollen is not toxic, even at large doses. It has traditionally been used as a permanent adjunct to the diet in both China and Korea. Government publications and the historical literature list no side effects.

Pine pollen should not be used for enhancing testosterone levels by adolescent men as it may interfere with the body's normal testosterone production. It should not be used by people with conditions of androgenic excess.

Herb/Drug Interactions: None known.

David's Lily (*Lilium davidii*)

Family: Liliaceae

Common Names: David's lily, chuan bai he (China).

Parts Used: For food, the root bulb. For androgen enhancement, primarily the anthers and pollen, however the whole flower is generally harvested and tinctured for use.

Habitat: This lily is native to China (Gansu, Henan, Hubei, Shaanxi, Sichuan, and Yunnan provinces), and the Indian subcontinent (states of Arunachal Pradesh and Manipur). Flower fanciers, however, have spread it around the world, and it is becoming naturalized everywhere. The plant grows three to five feet tall; the bright orange, black-spotted flowers grow singly or two to eight in a raceme. The plants like moist places in forests, forest margins, and grassy slopes, generally at elevations of 2,400 feet or higher. The plant is widely cultivated in China for its edible bulbs.

Cultivation: Usually from bulbs, like most members of this family.

Collection: Generally, the flowers are collected when they are mature and the pollen is well developed. The bulbs are usually harvested in autumn or winter. See the Scientific heading in this section for more on collecting this species for use in enhancing androgens in men.

Actions: Androgenic stimulant, relaxant.

Chemistry: Although extensive chemical profiles have been developed on many similar lilies, this species is very new to that type of examination. The chemistry of the lily family is complex, and steroidal compounds are common, including steroidal saponins, steroidal alkaloids, and now, in this species, steroidal hormones. All of these have impacts on human physiology.

Research on David's lily has found a number of integrin-like proteins, alpha-actinin-like proteins, F-actin, and G-actin. Beta-sitosterol, emodin, and stigmasterol are common in the plant. Of more interest for androgen supplementation is the research showing testosterone in the plant. Parts of the plant also contain estrogens, so the plant must be harvested at a specific time so that testosterone level is maximized.

About David's Lily: David's lily is widely cultivated in China for its edible bulbs. It has been an integral food plant there for millennia.

Native Americans, the Greeks and Romans, Europeans and the Chinese have all regularly eaten different species of lilies. Thoreau in his journal commented in July 1857 that he "dug some, and found a mass of bulbs pretty deep in the earth, two inches in diameter, looking and even tasting somewhat like raw green corn on the ear."

The lily family is large and contains 294 genera and some 4,500 species of herbs. Garlic and onion, *Alium* species, are members of the lily family, and like most lilies possess edible bulbs—what we call onions and garlic cloves. Like onions and garlic, the bulbs of lilies are pungent and are rarely eaten fresh. They are almost always cooked, usually baked or boiled. As with onions and garlic this softens the pungent nature of the plants and, for many types of edible lilies, makes them a delicious food.

Ayurvedic Use: Unknown as far as I can determine.

Traditional Chinese Medicine: The Chinese more often use the bulb as a nutritive and medicinal food than they do the flowers. Usually the root is baked or boiled, sometimes stuffed with a blend of pork, onions, and garlic.

In traditional Chinese practice the bulb has been used for coughs and sore throats, to clear the lungs, for low-grade fever, insomnia, restlessness, irritability, and for calming the spirit. Throughout Asia, the flower has been used as a relaxant for the nerves and a general, strengthening tonic.

Western Botanic Practice: David's lily is unknown in historical Western practice. However, other species of lily have extensive historical presence in Western botanic practice and have been used externally for bruises, boils, corns, burns, ulcers, inflammations, and softening hard skin. Internally they were used as anodynes (soothing pain), anti-epileptics, and relaxing nervines. Lily species are used as diuretics (promoting urine flow), for dropsy (i.e., the accumulation of water in the lower extremities from a poorly functioning heart), and for strengthening the heart.

Scientific Research: Modern analysis has found significant levels of testosterone in the anther (part that produces pollen) and pollen of David's lily, making it one of a handful of plants known, at this point, to possess testosterone as a constituent.

The testosterone in the plant is present in substantial quantities at only one time. That is when the anthers are producing pollen and just before pollen release. Levels of testosterone increase as the anthers' production of pollen comes into play then reach a maximum at anthesis (when the flower is in full bloom and the pollen is just about to be released for germination). After pollen shedding, testosterone levels drop rapidly. After pollination, as the testosterone levels drop, estrogen levels in the plant increase substantially. The plant is very time sensitive in this respect.

No clinical research has been done with this species of lily that I can find. I have used a tincture of the flowering plant and found it useful but with effects that were not as strong as those of pine pollen.

Availability: Woodland Essence, a natural medicine company, has been working on growing David's lily; I am not sure that they are producing sufficient quantities for production. The plant is primarily included in this book to try and stimulate more production of phytoandrogens by American herbal growers.

Suggested Dosage: The flowers at peak pollen production should be tinctured in alcohol. Tincture: ¼ teaspoon three times daily.

Side Effects and Contraindications: Begin with extremely low doses and work up. Some people have been known to experience extreme sensitivity and/or side effects to lily pollen. Try a small amount first to make sure that you are not sensitive. **If you have a history of allergies to pollen or severe reactions to bee stings, you should proceed with caution to make sure that your reactions do not extend to lily pollens.**

David's lily should not be used for enhancing testosterone by adolescent men as it may interfere with normal testosterone production by the body. Not for those with androgenic excess conditions.

Herb/Drug Interactions: None known.

Ginseng *(Panax ginseng)*

Family: Araliaceae

Common Names: Ginseng, panax, Asian ginseng, Chinese ginseng, Korean ginseng, Korean red, renshen (China).

Parts Used: Both the root and, sometimes, the above-ground plant. The above-ground plant, though weaker in its effects, does posses many of the same actions as the root. Use of the plant rather than the root is more ecologically sustainable. Ginseng is a perennial.

Habitat: Asian ginseng is native to China, Korea, and Russia, where it grows in regions very similar to the Appalachian and Ozark mountain ranges of the United States. Most of it is grown on the mountain slopes of China's northeastern ranges and in adjacent regions of Korea and Russia. Due to heavy medicinal use in China over thousands of years, the wild plant is exceptionally rare, and most Asian ginseng is now farm-raised. The older the roots, the stronger and more potent their chemistries.

Collection: Generally, ginseng roots are not harvested until at least the fifth year as research has shown that the ginsenoide content (perhaps the most important active constituent) of the roots becomes high at that time. The root also doubles in weight by the sixth year, making harvest at that time more profitable.

Actions: Adaptogenic, corticosteroidogenic, gonadotrophic, antifatigue, cardiotonic, hypoglycemic, hypothalamic tonic, pituitary stimulant, cognitive stimulant, central nervous system activator (thymoleptic), tonic and restorative, antitumor, immune stimulant, stomachic. Used in cases of weakness, loss of vitality, anemia, forgetfulness, and impotence.

Chemistry: The constituents of ginseng include twenty-eight different ginsenosides as well as polyacetylenes, alkaloids, polysaccharides, essential oils, fatty acids, steroids, amino acids, peptides, nucleotides, vitamins, choline, starch, pectins, and cellulose.

About Ginseng: The Asian species has been used for millennia in China; the American species by indigenous people for just as long. It is probably the only herb that nearly everyone in the United States has heard of. Often overused, overpriced, and oversold—still, when used for the right conditions, the results are exceptional.

Ayurvedic Use: A related species, *P. fruticosum*, has been used in Ayurvedic practice, but uncommonly.

Traditional Chinese Medicine: Chinese physicians have been using ginseng for at least two thousand years, the earliest mention occurring in medical texts in the first century. The Chinese process Asian ginseng in at least fifteen different ways, the two most common being "white" and "red" ginseng. "White" ginseng is the whole, carefully dried root. "Red" ginseng is processed by steaming the roots for three hours, drying them over a low fire, and compressing them into bricks of specific weight. Red ginseng is hard, brittle, almost glasslike, with a red, translucent look to it. When powdering for use as a tincture or to encapsulate, it sounds almost like broken glass in the blender. While possessing similar medicinal activities, there are slight differences between the two forms of Asian ginseng. Red, for example, shows more antioxidant activity. There are significant differences between American ginseng *(P. quinque-folius)* and Asian ginseng *(P. ginseng)*. The Chinese consider American ginseng more *yin* (female, cool, soft, yielding) and Asian ginseng more *yang* (male, hot, hard, aggressive). (Tienchi ginseng, on the other hand, is considered neutral, evenly balanced between yin and yang.) Scientific research has born this out in a number of ways, the most basic being that American ginseng contains the female hormone estradiol, an estrogen, while Asian ginseng does not.

Western Botanic Practice: Known but not generally used in early American practice. At that time, the emphasis was on American ginseng, *P. quinquefolia*. In Germany, Asian ginseng is now part of standard practice medicine and it is widely known throughout the Western countries. It often is used to promote male health and vitality. Too often, though, it is misused as a stimulant; it stimulates adrenal production through ginsenoside corticosteroid activation.

Scientific Research: More than three thousand scientific studies have been conducted on Asian ginseng over the past fifty years. The online database Medline alone lists 2,530 studies. In China, there are hundreds or thousands more that have not yet been translated into English. The kind of research that has been done has often differed depending on the country of origin. Steven Foster notes in *Herbal Emissaries* that, "Chinese researchers, as is the case with medicinal plants in general, have focused on *how* ginseng works, whereas western researchers focus on *if* it works . . . In Asia, the efficacy of an herb is already established in a cultural context. In the West we presuppose that traditional or folk uses have no rational scientific basis."[1]

Still, a great deal of important research has been done. As Foster goes on to note, Asian ginseng has been found to possess "radioprotective, antitumor, antiviral, and metabolic effects; antioxidant activities, nervous system and reproductive performance [effects]; effects on cholesterol and lipid metabolism; and endocrinological activity."[2] It is an adaptogen (increasing general strength and resistance to stress), an antifatigue, stimulates the adrenal cortex (corticosteroidogenic), supports skin regeneration, and has hypoglycemic activity. The science is not in doubt except to die-hard pharmaceutical and medical reductionists. What is most important are the studies supporting its use for balancing androgen shifts, for helping with many of the common problems men experience in middle age, especially reproductive problems.

European clinical studies have shown consistent shortening of reaction time to visual and auditory stimuli, heightened alertness, increased concentration, increased mental clarity, better grasp of abstract concepts, heightened visual and motor coordination, and stronger respiration after the use of Asian ginseng. Research shows clear activity for male reproductive systems. A few examples:

In one human trial with a saponin fraction (a constituent) of Asian ginseng in which volunteers took four grams per day for three months, researchers found that the men showed an increase of plasma testosterone, DHT, FSH (follicle stimulating hormone), LH (luteinizing hormone), number of sperm, and sperm motility. Luteinizing hormone stimulates the synthesis and secretion of testosterone into the bloodstream. Follicle stimulating hormone is critical for sperm production. It supports the function of the testes' Sertoli cells and thus stimulates the maturation and health of sperm. Russian researchers found in a number of clinical studies that ginseng is effective for impotence in both diabetic and non-diabetic populations. Two Russian clinical trials (of forty-four and twenty-seven men respectively) on the use of ginseng for impotence found that half the men recovered completely, the others improved.

In vivo studies (in living animals—rats and mice usually) have consistently shown increases in their levels of testosterone after powdered ginseng root was included in their diet, mixed with food. Both in vivo and in vitro (in lab glassware) studies show that ginseng and the ginsenosides present in Asian ginseng stimulate the release of luteinizing hormone as strongly as the luteinizing release hormone (called gonadotropin-releasing hormone, GnRH) produced by the body. This release of LH stimulates the male body to increase levels of testosterone. Numerous in vivo studies have shown that the herb stimulates sexual behavior, increases sperm counts and motility, and increases protein synthesis in the testes. The action appears to come primarily from a gonadotrophic action, that is it either mimics or stimulates the release of gonadotrophin (a sexually specific hormone) from the pituitary gland. In general, ginseng is considered to be a substance that stimulates the testes to produce more testosterone and sperm rather than being a substance that adds testosterone to the body.

Ginseng is also corticosteroidogenic, that is, it stimulates the release of cortisol and adrenaline from the adrenal glands. Too much of the herb can be, well, too much. This is why some of the side effects from overuse and overdosage occur. (See the Side Effects in this section.)

Suggested Dosage: Asian ginseng can be taken as tablets for one to nine grams per day or as a tincture. The tincture is prepared in a 1:5 mixture in 70 percent alcohol. The normal American dosage range is: Kirin (dark red): five to twenty drops per day. White: twenty to forty drops per day. Asians often consume it in much higher dosages.

Note: For androgen-replacement purposes, Asian ginseng should be used and *not* American ginseng. I generally prefer to combine Asian ginseng with Tienchi ginseng (see next listing) when using it for antifatigue actions. In such cases, I use a combination of Tienchi (tinctured 1:5, 70% alcohol) and Asian ginseng tinctures, half and half, one-third teaspoon per day in water.

Availability: Asian ginseng in many forms is widely available at health food stores and on the Internet.

Side Effects and Contraindications: Ginseng can be quite stimulating and should be used in small doses at first, and the dosage increased once you are used to it. It can sometimes cause hypertension, especially with large, sustained doses, and is contraindicated for those with extremely elevated blood pressure. It can be used with care in mild hypertension and with oversight in moderate hypertension. Sustained overuse can cause insomnia, sometimes heart palpitations, muscle tension, and headache. It may cause difficulty in sleeping if taken before bedtime.

Because ginseng affects androgen and testosterone levels, it should not be used by adolescent men. Not for use in androgenic excess conditions, not for use during pregnancy.

Herb/Drug Interactions: Ginseng should be avoided by people who are taking the drugs warfarin (Coumadin), phenelzine (Nardil), digoxin (Lanoxin), or haloperidol (Haldol). It should also be avoided by people who are taking hypoglycemic drugs, anticoagulants, or adrenal stimulants. Caution should be exercised in its use with MAO inhibitors. Ginseng may block the painkilling actions of morphine.

Tienchi Ginseng (Panax notoginseng, P. pseudoginseng var. notoginseng)

Family: Araliaceae

Common Names: Tienchi ginseng, san qi, tan qi

Habitat: This type of ginseng is native to northern India, Nepal, southern China, Vietnam, Thailand, and Japan. It likes the woods, much like American and Asian ginsengs. It, in fact, looks very similar to Asian ginseng.

Cultivation: From seed.

Collection: In the fall, after seeding.

Actions: Adaptogen, gonadotrophic, immune stimulant, blood tonic, antiarrhythmic, anti-inflammatory, antihemorrhagic, cardioprotective, hypocholesterolemic. Enhances sperm motility, stimulates production and release of nitric oxide and nitric oxide synthase. This latter action helps to expand coronary arteries to promote blood circulation and prevent blood clots. This also makes it a useful erection aid because erections are highly dependent on nitric oxide production.

Chemistry: Contains fourteen ginsenosides as well as flavonoids, B-sitosterol, daucosterol, numerous alkaloids, flavonol glycosides, various saponins, glycans, polysaccharide fraction DPG-3–2, peptides, (20)-protopanaxatriol, (20)-protopanaxadiol, panaxynal, quercitin, numerous polysaccharides, eight arasapogenins, and a number of vitamins and minerals, including A, B_6, and zinc. The arasapogenins are considered to be structurally similar to the ginsenosides and are sometimes referred to as notoginsenosides. The notoginsenosides are unique to tienchi ginseng, and their actions have not yet been explored fully.

About Tienchi Ginseng: Although tienchi and Asian ginseng do have many ginsenosides in common, ginseng has more, about twenty-eight to tienchi's fourteen. Tienchi, as well, has its own unique compounds, the notoginsenosides. So, while there is some overlap in function, each plant has a unique chemical profile that produces unique actions in the body. I like tienchi for men because of its impacts on blood circulation, the heart, nitric oxide production, sperm production and motility, and erectile function.

In traditional Chinese use, tienchi ginseng has been known primarily for its actions in the cardiovascular system. However, its ginsenosides as well as the notoginsenosides that are unique to tienchi ginseng have steroidal-like impacts on male physiology. Many of them are considered to be gonadotrophic, that is they stimulate the testes to produce more testosterone and sperm. Sperm motility is enhanced, and the body produces more nitric oxide and nitric oxide synthase, which is an enzyme that acts in the body to produce nitric oxide. Nitric oxide is involved in many physiological processes, including blood pressure control, neurotransmission, learning, and memory. In high concentrations it acts as a defensive cytotoxin—part of the immune response to disease. Nitric oxide is especially important for men's erections, it works to stimulate blood vessel expansion and blood flow in the heart and penis.

One of the reasons the herb works so well for preventing and cor-

recting heart conditions is that it stimulates the proliferation of endothelial progenitor cells in the blood. A form of stem cells, endothelial progenitor cells are formed in the bone marrow. One of their main functions
is to repair damage to the lining of blood vessels. The higher the count of
these cells in the blood, the lower the incidence of disease. The number
of endothelial progenitor cells tends to be low in people with multivessel
disease, diabetes, a history of heart attack, and atherosclerosis. Tienchi
ginseng's stimulation of these cells is significant.

Tienchi ginseng can be purchased as a whole dried root, a sliced
dried root, or a prepared root. The prepared root is generally small,
black, and marble-sized, with the same glasslike properties as kirin red
ginseng. I have generally used the prepared root to enhance health, vitality, and male reproduction. The whole and sliced roots are sometimes
used in China as a food, generally steamed. The steamed root is sometimes dried and encapsulated as well. In Chinese practice, the steamed
root is considered to be more of a system tonic, while the unsteamed
root is considered better for treating the blood.

Ayurvedic Use: A related species, *P. fruticosum,* has been used in
Ayurvedic practice but is uncommon.

Traditional Chinese Medicine: A relative newcomer to Chinese practice,
tienchi ginseng has only been in use for five hundred years. Its primary
use is for the blood, heart, and circulatory system. The herb is used primarily for blood stasis and improper blood conditions. It is specific for
serious bleeding and traumatic shock.

Western Botanic Practice: Unknown until recent introduction from China
and Japan, it is beginning to be well established in Western practice.

Scientific Research: Compared with Asian ginseng, tienchi is a relative
newcomer to scientific study. There are only four or five hundred studies
on record, about 240 of them in the online Medline database. However,
examination of the plant has found the same ginsenosides (though fewer
of them) as those in Asian ginseng.

In hundreds of studies, researchers have consistently found that ginsenosides have active pharmacological effects in the cardiovascular, endocrine, and central nervous systems. Ginsenosides have been found to have anticarcinogenic effects through a number of different mechanisms—either by direct cytotoxic effects or by induction of differentiation and inhibition of metastasis. Ginsenosides and notoginsenosides also have a number of specific actions in the central nervous system and brain. Ginsenoside Rg1, for example, modulates neurotransmission and prevents chemically-induced memory deficits by increasing cholinergic activity. This same compound also has immunomodulating effects, increasing both humoral and cell-mediated immune responses.

Scores of in vivo studies in China have found tienchi to have profound positive effects on the cardiovascular system, especially in the treatment of myocardial infarction, angina, and narrowing of blood vessels. Further tests found that it shortens blood-clotting time and is a strong anti-inflammatory.

Clinical trials of patients with coronary artery disease found significant improvements with use of the herb, angina decreased in frequency and intensity. Other clinical trials treating hemoptysis (blood from the lungs) were effective as well, with interior bleeding completely arrested. Both hematuria (blood clots resulting from head injury) and intraocular hemorrhage have responded to the herb in clinical trials. The herb is exceptionally good if there are blood clots from traumatic injury.

Some concern has been raised in the use of this herb as an androgenic supplement because of the presence of ginsenoside Rg1, which is a tremendously potent phytoestrogen. Although that compound *is* present in the plant, the whole plant itself, when used as a supplement, does not produce estrogenic outcomes because there are scores of other compounds involved, not just this isolated constituent. There is a synergistic effect that occurs when the herb is taken whole.

Clinical use has been consistent. The herb enhances energy levels, increases mental clarity, helps with libido, erection, sperm motility, and vitality.

Suggested Dosage: 1:5 tincture, thirty drops (1.5 mL or ⅜ tsp.) three times daily. In severe depletion conditions the dose may be increased to twice that amount but side effects should be monitored. **Note:** For male health, as an antifatigue agent, and testosterone enhancement, I prefer to combine tienchi and Asian ginseng. I generally use a combination of Tienchi (tinctured 1:5, 70% alcohol) and Asian ginseng tinctures, half and half, taking ⅓ teaspoon per day in water.

Side Effects and Contraindications: Tienchi ginseng can produce allergic reactions in a small percentage of users. Generally these manifest as some sort of rash—hives, red papules, skin itching, flushed skin. Very rarely, there can be mild anaphylaxis, abdominal pain or swelling, and diarrhea. These reactions are uncommon, with only about nineteen reported instances in the literature out of millions of users.

High doses of tienchi ginseng can cause nervousness, sleeplessness, anxiety, breast pain, headaches, high blood pressure, insomnia, and restlessness. The plant is a corticosteroidogenic herb, that is, it stimulates the production of catabolic steroids such as adrenaline and cortisol by the adrenal glands.

The herb should be discontinued at least seven days prior to surgery because ginseng can lower blood glucose level and act as a blood thinner. It should not be used during pregnancy because some of its constituents can cross from breast milk into nursing children. (These conditions correct upon discontinuance of the herb.) It should not be used by adolescent men because it can interfere with the body's normal testosterone production. It should not be used by people with conditions of androgenic excess.

Herb/Drug Interactions: Do not use with blood thinning agents, warfarin (may decrease effectiveness). It may and probably will increase the effects of amphetamine-like stimulants, including caffeine. Do not use with haloperidol, an antipsychotic, it may exaggerate its effects. Tienchi may block the effects of morphine, and its use with MAO inhibitors such as phenelzine may cause symptoms such as headaches, manic episodes, and tremulousness.

Eleuthero aka Siberian Ginseng *(Eleutherococcus senticosus, Acanthopanax senticosus)*

Family: Araliaceae

Common Names: Siberian ginseng, eleuthero, ci-wu-jia (China), devil's shrub, touch-me-not (Russia).

Parts Used: The cortex (outer layer) of the root, the whole root, and the bark.

Cultivation: From seeds.

Collection and Habitat: Siberian ginseng, a persistent, aggressive shrub from three to fifteen feet in height, grows throughout parts of China, Russia, Korea, and even a bit in the northern islands of Japan. It is covered with spines and has an aggressive, intimidating presence that has given rise to some of its common Russian names—touch-me-not and devil's shrub.

Due to its popularity as a medicinal, it is undergoing heavy planting in the United States and has begun to escape captivity. Soon it will be, like a number of important medicinals, among them Japanese knotweed, a naturalized, aggressive weed with qualities unknown to those it irritates.

The bark is generally harvested in late summer or fall; the roots when the plant goes dormant in late fall. In China only the cortex, or outer layer, of the root is used while in Russia they use the whole root. In the United States we tend to follow the Russian lead and use the whole root. When purchased, the root usually has been cut and sifted or powdered to industry standards. Adulteration of Chinese imports is a problem. North American-grown eleuthero is generally more reliable.

Actions: Mild androgen, adaptogen, antistressor, immune tonic (or stimulant depending on preparation), immune-potentiator (increases nonspecific immunity), immunoadjuvant, adrenal tonic, increases non-specific resistance against a number of pathogens, cardiotonic, antirheumatic, increases cerebral blood flow, dilates blood vessels, and is a MAO inhibitor. It is especially indicated for people with pale unhealthy skin, lassitude, and depression.

Chemistry: Thirteen different eleutherosides, six different senticosides, polysaccharides pes-A and pes-B, alpha maltose, beta-carotene, beta-maltose, beta-sitosterol, betulinic acid, caffeic acid, caffeic acid ethyl ester, coniferyl aldehyde, copper, coumarin-x, d-galactose, d-clucose, caucosterin, eleutherans, eleutherococcal, eo, glycans, isofraxidin, oleanolic acid, pectic, resin, saponins, sesamin, sinapylalcohol, sucrose, syringaresinol-diglycoside, syringin, and vitamin E.

About Eleuthero: Although used in China for several thousand years, eleutherococcus (or Siberian ginseng as many people still prefer to call it) was used primarily by the Chinese for spasms. It was brought to prominence as an immune tonic and adaptogen as a result of intensive Russian research in the latter half of the twentieth century (and has now traveled back to China as an adaptogenic herb).

Ayurvedic Use: Unknown.

Traditional Chinese Medicine: Eleuthero has been used in Chinese medicine for over 2,000 years. It is considered good for vital energy, strengthening the spleen and kidney, for deficiency of yang in the spleen and kidney, and for stabilizing energy.

Western Botanic Practice: Unknown until the Russian research brought it to prominence in the late twentieth century. Now it is a staple in the Western herbal pharmacopoeia.

Scientific Research: Eleuthero contains two known androgenic substances: eleutheroside-B-1 and eleutheroside-E. Preliminary work on the effects of the herb on male reproductive health has shown that it increases the weight of prostate and seminal vesicles in castrated rats (118% and 70%, respectively) and that it also prevents the atrophy of the prostate and seminal vesicles if given to rats before castration. Essentially, eleuthero can keep levels of male androgens high enough that even when the primary source of testosterone is lost through castration, the rest of the sexual organs remain normal.

A number of clinical trials have shown significant immune-enhancing activity, including significant increases in immunocompetent cells, specifically T-lymphocytes (helper/inducers, cytotoxic and natural killer cells). Tests of the herb have repeatedly shown that it increases the ability of human beings to withstand adverse conditions, increases mental alertness, and improves performance. People taking the herb consistently report fewer illnesses than those who do not take the herb. Part of its power is its ability to act as a tonic stimulant on the adrenal glands. It normalizes adrenal activity and moves adrenal action away from a cortisol/catabolic dynamic to a DHEA/anabolic orientation. Basically, this reduces stress and normalizes physiological functioning throughout the body.

In one Russian clinical trial, 2,100 healthy adults were given the herb and found to better handle stressful conditions. They showed increased ability to perform physical labor, withstand motion sickness, and work with speed and precision despite loud surroundings. Their ability to accurately proofread documents increased, and they more readily adapted to diverse physical stresses, including high altitudes, heat, and low-oxygen environments.

Another Russian study of 13,000 auto workers found that those who took the herb developed 40 percent fewer respiratory infections than normal for their group.

Other studies have found that the herb heightens mental alertness, improves concentration, and boosts the transmission of nerve impulses in the brain.

Eleutherococcus senticosus and a related species, *E. chiisanensis,* have been found to be strongly antihepatotoxic and hepatoprotective in vivo against CCL4-induced hepatotoxicity. (In other words, they strongly protect the liver from damage by toxins and chemicals.) Additionally, eleuthero has been found to be a hepatoregenerator, significantly stimulating liver regeneration in animals with portions of their livers surgically removed.

Because the herb is a MAO inhibitor, it is also useful in depression, a condition that often accompanies a severely depleted immune system and chronic liver disease.

These overall effects make eleuthero a good herb for men experiencing low libido, loss of energy, or problems with androgen levels in middle age.

Suggested Dosage: Most of the Russian studies were conducted using a 1:1 tincture with 30 to 33 percent alcohol. The Russians generally dosed 2 to 16 mL one to three times each day for sixty days with a two- to three-week rest period in between. Ill patients received less, 0.5 to 6 mL one to three times per day for three days then a two- to three-week rest period in between. At these kinds of dosages, Russian researchers saw responses within a few days or even hours of administration. Some of the American companies that utilize the Russian approach for tincturing also like to standardize their formulas for specific eleutheroside content. Tinctures that, like the Russian formulations, are 1:1 or 1:2 are black in color (in contrast to 1:5 formulations, which are golden). Remember to look for a black tincture to ensure that it is a 1:1 or 1:2 formulation.

I suggest the product made by Herb Pharm, which is the only company I know of that actually exceeds the Russian specifications. Their formula is a 2:1 tincture (two parts herb to one part liquid) rather than a 1:1 tincture. For the first thirty to sixty days: one teaspoon of the tincture three times daily, the last dose occurring by 4 p.m. This amount can be increased if necessary. Discontinue the herb for two weeks. Repeat the course if necessary. If symptoms decrease after using the Russian formulation and immune function seems better, the type of formulation used can change to either an encapsulated form or a 1:5 alcohol/water tincture (one part herb to five parts liquid). Both these formulations are weaker than the Russian approach.

As an encapsulated form, I suggest a 450 mg capsule of a formulation standardized to 0.8 percent eleutherosides B&E, particularly Nature's Way capsules, which contain 250 mg of standardized extract and 200 mg of the whole herb. Take two capsules four times daily for the eight to twelve months of treatment.

Alternate Preparations: Although I prefer the Russian formulation for androgen enhancement and to treat severe chronic diseases like Lyme borreliosis and chronic fatigue, I generally use and prefer a weaker tincture for people with general weakness and fatigue, as do many American herbalists. People with these conditions should take a full dropper (30 drops) of a 1:5, 60-percent alcohol tincture one to three times each day for up to a year. In my experience, this dosage and use pattern is less stimulating to the system and the long-term effects are better. The body gradually uses the herb to build itself up over time, the herb acting more as a long-term tonic and rejuvenative than an active stimulant. With this type of tincture, it is not necessary to stop every one to two months, nor have I seen any of the side effects that can occur with the stronger Russian formulation.

The Chinese, much less given to tincturing anyway, use 4.5 to 27 grams, often as a decoction or powder.

Tinctures, tablets, and capsules are widely available at health food stores and on the Internet.

For Increasing Androgen Levels: If your libido and energy levels are low, then the Russian formulation is going to be the most effective form of the herb to take. The Herb Pharm product is the best for this.

Side Effects and Contraindications: Eleuthero is, in general, completely nontoxic and the Russians have reported taking exceptionally large doses for up to twenty years with no adverse reactions. The lower strength 1:5 formula rarely shows any side effects at all, most side effects refer to the 1:1 or 1:2 formulas and even for these formulations most people experience no side effects.

Contraindicated in pregnancy. Insomnia and hyperactivity can occur with use of the stronger Russian formulation especially when taken in large doses, with caffeine, or late in the afternoon or evening. A very small number of people have experienced transient diarrhea. May temporarily increase blood pressure in some people. This tends to drop to normal within a few weeks. Caution should be exercised for people with very high blood pressure especially if combined with other hypertensives such as licorice. With extreme overuse: tension and insomnia.

Herb/Drug Interactions: 1:1 or 1:2 formulas—should not be used by people who are taking digoxin or sedatives, especially barbiturates such as pentobarbital.

Nettle Root *(Urtica dioica)*

Family: Urticaceae

Parts Used: To increase testosterone levels and for prostate health, the root; for gout, the plant; for arthritis, the plant and its "sting;" and for kidney health, the seeds.

Collection and Habitat: Nettles grow throughout the world, the root can be harvested at any time but is often picked in the spring before the nettles and their stings are much advanced. The plant is usually harvested in early to late spring, almost always prior to seeding. The seeds are harvested when ripe.

Actions: Male sexual tonic, nutritive, astringent, diuretic, antirheumatic, antigout, sex hormone binding globulin (SHBG) inhibitor, antiaromatasic.

Chemistry: Nettle contains a number of powerful chemical constituents. They are either unique to this plant, unique in these quantities, or unique in these combinations. Of note are histamine, formic acid, acetylcholine, 5–hydroxytryptamine, various glucoquinones, and the aromatase inhibitor (10E,12Z)-9-hydroxy-10,12-octadecadienoic acid. Nettle is also exceptionally high in many vitamins and minerals, including zinc, and contains more protein than any other land plant.

The constituents of nettle are extensive: 2-methylhepten-(2)-on-(6), 5-hydroxytryptamine, acetic acid, acetophenone, acetylcholine, alpha-tocopherol, aluminum arsenic, ascorbic acid, beta-carotene, betaine, boron, bromine, butyric acid, cadmium, caffeic acid, calcium, carbohydrates, cellulose, chlorine, chlorophyll, choline, chromium, cobalt, copper, fat, ferulic acid, fluorine, folacin, formic acid, glycerol, histamine, iron, coproporphyrin, lead, lecithin, linoleic acid, linolenic acid, lycopene, magnesium, manganese, mercury, molybdenum, mucilage, niacin, nickel, nitrogen, oleic acid, p-coumaric acid, palmitic acid, pantothenic acid, phosphorus, potassium, protein, protoporphyrin, riboflavin, rubidium, scopoletic, selenium, serotonin, sfa, silicon, sitosterol, sitosterol-glucoside, sodium, sulfur, thiamin, tin, violananthin, xanthophyll-epoxide, and zinc.

About Nettle and Nettle Root: A native of Europe and the United States, nettle has been extensively used throughout its native ranges as a primary part of herbal care for millennia. Often one of the first plants to be available in early spring, it has had a primary place in folk practice as one of the most reliable spring tonics and healing plants known.

Ayurvedic Use: Uncommon and not a part of traditional Ayurvedic practice due to its being mostly a European herb. It has been used in India only after its introduction from Europe. Although it is used rarely, its applications are similar to those of European folk practice.

Traditional Chinese Medicine: Not a part of traditional Chinese medicine.

Western Botanic Practice: Has been used since the dawn of time.

Scientific Research: Of most importance in helping raise testosterone levels, nettle root has been found to inhibit the binding of dihydrotestosterone (DHT) to sex hormone binding globulin (SHBG), in human trial thus keeping body levels of androgens higher. A general inhibition of SHBG binding has been found in other human studies and in a great many in vitro studies with human cells. Nettle root also possesses strong antiaromatase action, thus interfering with the conversion of testosterone to estradiol. This has been found to occur in the human placenta, in animal studies, and in vitro. Nettle root is specifically indicated if you suffer both BPH and low testosterone levels.

Nettle root possesses powerful tonic actions for the male prostate. It has been used to treat both BPH and prostatitis in at least thirty clinical studies. Participants in the studies ranged from as few as twenty men to as many as 5,400. In men with Stage I to III BPH, nettle root consistently reduced nocturia (nighttime urination), improved urine stream, decreased urine remaining in the bladder after urination, and decreased prostate size. Its use also resulted in significantly lower scores on the International Prostate Symptom Score questionnaire, which rates the degree of negative impacts on urination from prostate inflammation in seven areas plus overall quality of life. A number of the trials were double-blind, placebo-controlled, crossover studies.

A few examples:

From 61 to 83 percent of 5,492 men who used 1200 mg of nettle root daily for three to four months found significant relief from BPH symptoms.

In twenty-six men who used 1200 mg of a nettle root daily, prostate volume decreased in 54 percent and residual volume of urine in seventy-five percent.

Seventy-nine men who used 600 mg of nettle root per day for sixty-eight weeks (sixteen months) found that urine flow significantly increased and urination time significantly decreased.

Twenty patients who used a combination of nettle root and saw palmetto in a placebo-controlled, randomized, double-blind trial found that their flow rate significantly improved over placebo. Their International Prostate Symptom Score results declined from 18.6 to 11.1 and with continued use further declined to 9.8. The study found that continued use of the herbs increased prostate shrinkage over time, improving prostate health the longer they are used. The same study compared 489 men with others using finasteride (Proscar) over a forty-eight week period and found that International Prostate Symptom Score results dropped similarly in both groups but that the men using herbal extracts had fewer side effects.

Needle biopsies were taken in a number of studies to discover exactly what was happening to the prostate in men taking nettle root. Researchers found that nettle root reduced the activity of the smooth muscle cells in the prostate, caused shrinkage of the epithelial or glandular tissue, and increased epithelial secretions.

Nettle root has been found to be consistently anti-inflammatory (both to the prostate and other tissues), to inhibit production of SHBG, to inhibit the binding of DHT to SHBG, and to be antiaromatasic (inhibiting the conversion of testosterone to estradiol).

Suggested Dosage: The dosage varies depending on what kind of nettle preparation you buy.

The capsule dosage ranges from 300 to 1200 mg per day of nettle root for three to twelve months in the majority of the clinical trials. This generally is the preferred form for male reproductive health.

The tincture dosage range is from 30 to 150 drops (1–5 full drop-pers, ⅜ to 2 tsp.) daily of a 45 percent alcohol/water tincture for one to twelve months.

Make sure in buying capsules and tinctures that you get prepara-tions made from nettle root and *not* the plant because each is used to treat different conditions.

Side Effects and Contraindications: Mild side effects have occasionally been reported with the root, usually mild gastrointestinal upset. With the plant, only mild side effects have been noted, including skin afflic-tions such as rashes and mild swelling. The Physicians Desk Reference for Herbal Medicines lists a contraindication for the plant in cases of people with fluid retention from reduced cardiac or renal action. No contraindications are noted for the root.

Herb/Drug Interactions: There is a slight possibility that the use of nettle root can decrease the effects of anticoagulants.

Tribulus *(Tribulus terrestris)*

Family: Zygophyllaceae

Common Names: Tribulus, puncture vine, caltrop, cat's head, devil's thorn, devil's weed, goat head, ji li (China), gokhru (India), and a variety of local insulting names and epithets, depending on location and degree of damage to persons and property.

Parts Used: Usually the dried fruit is used, especially to enhance fertility, although the leafy plant and root are also effective and sometimes used medicinally as well.

Collection and Habitat: Tribulus is a relatively small, low, weedy, shrubby, vine, sort-of-innocuous, nasty-looking plant that is widely distributed nat-urally in Asia throughout the tropics and subtropics, including Africa and Australia. It has also, happily, naturalized throughout much of the world, especially in California and parts of the American West. The root may be picked at any time, the plant when mature, and the fruit when ripe.

Actions: Reproductive and urinary tonic, antilithic (prohibiting or reducing kidney stones), hypotensive, diuretic, demulcent, aphrodisiac, DHEA production stimulant, and cardiac tonic for angina pectoris. The stems are considered to be a reliable astringent.

Chemistry: The fruits contain a number of alkaloids and saponins, some of them steroidal in nature. A number of researchers think that compounds they have dubbed furostanol saponins are the active constituents. Time will tell, as the plant is loaded with active compounds. These include beta-sitosterol, campesterol, 25-D-spirosta-3,5-diene, aspartic acid, astragalin, calcium, chlorogenic, cracillin, daucosterol, desoxydiogenin, diosgenin, diosgin, gitogenin, glutamic acid, harman, harmine, hecogenin, kaempferol, kaempferol-3-0-glucoside, kaempferol-3-0-rutinoside, kaempferol-3-beta-d-glucoside, linoleic acid, neogitogenin, neohecogenin glucopyranoside, oleic acid, palmitic acid, protodioscin, quercetin, ruscogenin, rutin, saponoside-c, stearic acid, stigmasterol, terrestroside, tribuloside, tribulosin, and so on.

About Tribulus: Tribulus is considered a noxious weed by many Westerners, especially those occupying Australia. Asians seem more understanding, perhaps because of their long use of the herb in traditional medicine. Called puncture vine for a reason, the spiny seeds are ferocious and nearly impossible to remove once embedded. They can puncture feet, animal paws, and bicycle tires with equal impunity.

Ayurvedic Use: In traditional Ayurvedic and Unani practice, tribulus has been used for at least three thousand years for the treatment of kidney stones, to increase urine and semen production, and as an aphrodisiac.

Traditional Chinese Medicine: Used for some four hundred years in Chinese medicine, tribulus is used for headaches, vertigo, dizziness, red, swollen and painful eyes, eye tearing, skin lesions, itching and hives, impotence, spermatorrhea, and pain in the loins.

Western Botanic Practice: Westerners, coming along some three millennia later than practitioners in India and using an entirely different approach, are finding the plant useful for: reducing kidney stones, increasing urine production, increasing semen production and sperm motility, and increasing sexual drive and performance. The actions of tribulus on the mucous membranes of the urinary tract are toning, astringent, and antibacterial, similar in action to that of buchu and uva ursi, two other well-known urinary system tonics.

Scientific Research: Studies have shown that tribulus increases serum levels of luteinizing hormone (LH), leading to higher levels of testosterone. Other studies have found consistently increased sexual drive in men who take the herb. And yet others showed a significant increase of DHEAS (a slightly different form of DHEA) in men's urine after they used tribulus for three weeks. Overall, tribulus is a useful herb for increasing testosterone levels and rebalancing the androgen/estrogen ratio. It is specifically indicated if you suffer from low sperm count and low sperm motility (or erectile dysfunction) and low serum testosterone levels. The herb shows a profound impact on male reproductive health, especially sperm production and motility.

Clinical study has found that from 50 to 80 percent of people using standardized preparations of tribulus experience significantly improved sperm production and motility. One study noted that taking five hundred milligrams of tribulus three times a day for sixty days significantly increased sperm production for men diagnosed with idiopathic oligozoospermia (men who show no sperm in the semen from no discernable cause). Libido, erection, ejaculation, and orgasm all increased significantly for 80 percent of the men. Another, double-blind, placebo-controlled trial showed significant increases in sperm motility with corresponding decreases in immotile sperm. Numerous other studies have shown similar outcomes. Tribulus has been found to increase the production of LH, follicle stimulating hormone (FSH), and, interestingly, estradiol in women and testosterone in men but not vice versa. This indicates it is a general reproductive system adaptogen and tonic, rather than specific to gender. Follicle stimulating hormone is critical for sperm production. It supports the testes' Sertoli cells and stimulates the production and maturation of sperm. A listing of relevant studies can be found in the Tribulus section in the Bibliography.

Suggested Dosage: A number of researchers and clinicians feel that the herb should be standardized for what they call furostanol saponin content, and some companies do so between 40 and 45 percent furostanols. It is available under a number of brand names: Tribestan, Trilovin, Libilov, and so on, and can be easily found on the Internet and in many health food stores. The usual dosage for infertility is between 250 and 500 milligrams three times a day for two to three months (or as directed).

The fruits themselves may also be used (as they traditionally have been for millennia) as an infusion or decoction of the powdered fruits, 1.5 to 3 grams daily.

Side Effects and Contraindications: Sheep and goats do not respond well to the herb. Occasionally the plant can be infected with a fungus while in storage. This can be avoided if you harvest the plant yourself or if you buy a commercial, standardized preparation. The plant itself is not known to cause adverse reactions in people, and there are no known contraindications for use.

Herb/Drug Interactions: None known.

5 SUPPLEMENTS TO INCREASE TESTOSTERONE LEVELS

What is the collateral damage of the pharmacist's pipette?

DALE PENDELL

Pharmaceutical manufacturers were some of the original creators of supplemental androgens, now commonly known as anabolic steroids. Initially, there was tremendous excitement among physicians and athletes (weight lifters and muscle builders especially) and pharmaceutical steroids were widely prescribed. Unfortunately, many of the people who used the synthetic steroids (testosterone propionate, testosterone cypionate, testosterone enanthate, testosterone undecanoate, and so on) became quite ill some years later, some dying from liver disease or cancer. The negative impacts from these artificial steroids are the result of how they are produced.

As with many synthetic pharmaceuticals, the natural molecule, testosterone in this instance, is altered just enough (toward the direction of being longer-lasting, more assimilatable, or more potent) so that a patent can be obtained. What manufacturers basically do is tack on an extra molecule to the testosterone molecule. As with all synthetic pharmaceuticals, the human body takes what it knows from its long evolutionary history (in this case, the testosterone molecule), separates it from any alien molecular structures, uses the testosterone, and is left with the problem of getting rid of the remaining molecular fragments. These leftover molecular fragments are often processed in the liver and are the source of the toxicity associated with anabolic steroids. As Jonathan Wright, M.D., coauthor of *Maximize Your Vitality and Potency for Men Over 40,* comments: "Call them what you will, hormone-like drugs are most definitely not hormones, and they *never* work exactly like natural hormones."[1]

Because of the toxicity of artificial hormones, many people began exploring the use of natural hormones that do not possess the toxicity of synthetic anabolic steroidal drugs. The alternatives they found were *natural* prohormonal substances, which synthetic drugs are not. Unfortunately, most of these natural androgenic supplements, *identical* to the hormones produced in the human body, were outlawed in the United States in January 2005 with the passage of the Anabolic Steroid Control Act—supposedly to protect children from buying them. Despite their exceptional safety record, the outcry over prohormone use in sports stimulated a more aggressive than normal form of puritanitis (spasming of the Puritan reflex) in the Congress and presidency.

Of the following supplements: pregnenolone, DHEA, zinc, vitamin B_5, androstenedione, and DHT, only the first four are still legal as individual supplements in the United States. Information on androstenedione is included because it is one of the constituents found in pine pollen and it makes sense to understand what the constituent does for male health. Information on DHT is included because of the bad press it has received. The negative information on DHT, its relation to prostate enlargement and male health in general, that is prevalent in the U.S. culture today, is incorrect. This is a small attempt to begin rectifying that problem. Like cholesterol, DHT is being demonized, and will eventually be understood to be critically important in male health. In fact, DHT suppressors can, like cholesterol suppressors, cause more harm than good.

The supplements listed in this chapter have all been found to increase testosterone levels in the blood and help restore a healthy androgen/estrogen ratio. Some men prefer to use testosterone in the form of injections, patches, implants, creams, or sublingual pills, rather than testosterone precursors or natural androgens such as the ones that follow. If you would like more information on that approach, the two best books are *Maximize Your Vitality and Potency for Men Over 40* and Eugene Shippen and William Fryer's *The Testosterone Syndrome*.

In seeking out natural androgenic supplements, you should make sure you are getting pure pharmaceutical-grade supplements and nothing else. Many of these supplements are made from the Mexican wild yam *(Dioscorea spp.)*, and some confusion has arisen as a result. Some people recommend the use of wild yam itself as a steroidal precursor, however, the human body cannot alter the compounds in wild yam into testosterone or any testosterone precursors. Wild yam is completely ineffective as a "natural" hormone for men or women unless its compounds have been extracted and chemically altered or processed in a laboratory.

Supplements to Increase Testosterone Levels

Pregnenolone, 50–100 mg day

DHEA, 25–50 mg day

Zinc, 20–60 mg day

Vitamin B$_5$, 100–500 mg daily

Pregnenolone

Pregnenolone is the first metabolite of cholesterol—the first thing cholesterol is made into. Thus, it is the primary steroid hormone (in both women and men) from which all the others are made. For this reason, it is sometimes called a prohormone or the "mother" steroid. Despite its being recognized as an important steroidal metabolite of cholesterol, there hasn't been much research on pregnenolone raising androgen levels. Although it is commonly used by many people for that purpose, it is not known whether in fact it does so. The primary effect of pregnenolone that is widely agreed upon is that it appears to enhance mental functioning. It acts as a mood elevator and a mild sharpener of the memory and senses. One placebo-controlled trial has shown that taking fifty milligrams of pregnenolone per day will reduce general fatigue levels by half and that the reduction continues for at least two weeks. In airline pilots, fifty milligrams of pregnenolone has been found to significantly enhance performance. It has also shown beneficial effects for arthritis and Alzheimer's disease.

Pregnenolone was also used extensively in the 1950s for treating collagen diseases such as lupus, rheumatoid arthritis, ankylosing spondylitis, and scleroderma that affect the collagen in bones and connective tissues. Numerous clinical trials and studies have shown its effectiveness for these kinds of conditions with decreases in pain, more mobility, and less stiffness.

Suggested Dosage: The dosage generally should be five to fifty milligrams per day. Anecdotal evidence has reported that doses as high as five hundred milligrams per day may in some instances help with the extreme memory loss and mental fatigue (brain fog) that occurs from Chronic Fatigue Syndrome. This is not usually recommended because of pregnenolone's side effects.

Side Effects: Hyperalertness, irritability, mood changes, headaches, and insomnia sometimes occur, especially at high doses. *This can be exacerbated markedly by coffee intake.* Reduce dosage or discontinue the supplement if these side effects occur.

Dehydroepiandrosterone (DHEA)

DHEA has been studied intensely in the past ten to twenty years. At least ten books about DHEA have been published, with scores more that discuss DHEA along with other supplements. While DHEA itself is only a mild androgen, it is the precursor for androstenedione and androstenediol, which are the precursors of testosterone, making it essential for testosterone production. In addition, it has shown significant positive effects on human health in almost every organ system in the body.

DHEA is the most abundant steroid in the human bloodstream; most of it (about 70 percent) is made from DHEA sulfate (DHEAS). The body essentially stores DHEA in a more stable form as DHEAS and converts it to DHEA (and then other androgens) whenever it is needed. Like testosterone, both DHEA and DHEAS levels decline over time, but much more quickly. Levels of DHEA reach a peak around a man's twenty-fifth year, then decline by about 2 percent per year; by age eighty, there is only 10 to 15 percent of age twenty levels. Normal levels of DHEA in the blood are 250 to 650 micrograms per deciliter (about one tenth of a quart) of blood; DHEAS levels are five hundred to one thousand times higher. (DHEAS and DHEA can be considered interchangeable when talking about their health effects.) People with levels of DHEA below 100 micrograms per deciliter consistently show higher levels of cancer, heart disease, diabetes, and arthritis.

Most DHEA is synthesized in the adrenal glands, about 10 percent is made in the testes, while the rest is made in the brain, the heart, and the liver. Because of its synthesis in the brain, DHEA is also considered to be a neurosteroid, having potent impacts on the central nervous system and brain function.

Contrary to earlier medical perspectives, it is now known that the brain can synthesize sex steroids. To some extent, this occurs in response to erotic imagery. Smell, also, can lead to increases. This has been demonstrated in rats where the smell of a female in estrous leads to significant increases of DHEA in the hypothalamus. (Men, exposed to tiny quantities of the sweat of a woman who is sexually excited, also experience increases in testosterone production.) However, the brain creates potent androgens for many reasons other than sex. They also play crucial roles in memory and neural activity in the brain and central nervous system, and DHEA is a crucial precursor to the creation of both androgens and estrogens in the brain.

DHEA is also metabolized in peripheral tissues to more active androgens and these levels never appear in the bloodstream. Basically, peripheral tissues in the human body make more active androgens from DHEA whenever they need them. Peripheral tissues in the body normally contain all the enzymes necessary to convert DHEA to androstenedione and then to testosterone. This allows potent androgens to be used at the site where they are most needed and perhaps explains how DHEA is able to affect so many different parts of the body. In essence, the androgens synthesized from DHEA exert their effects within the same cells where synthesis takes place, and these synthesized androgens are rarely released into general blood circulation, thus never showing up in blood tests. The parts of the body that are engaging in androgen synthesis are essentially using an extremely sophisticated biofeedback loop to determine exactly what levels of androgens are necessary and then making exactly what they need from the DHEA that normally circulates in the body. At least 30 to 50 percent of the total androgens in men are synthesized in peripheral tissues in just this way. The enzymes that are used for this androgen synthesis (or metabolic conversion) and the basic androgenic precursors, especially DHEA, are, thus, absolutely necessary for overall health.

Because DHEA can be converted to the estrogens estrone and estradiol, some people feel that DHEA is a potential problem when used in androgen-replacement therapy. No research has found this to occur; estrogen levels in men consistently remain unaffected by DHEA intake. For example, one study of sixty- to seventy-year-old men who received intramuscular DHEA injections showed increased levels of DHEA and androstenedione in their blood. *No change was found in their levels of estrone and estradiol.* Even with extremely high oral dosing of 1,600 milligrams per day in young, healthy men, levels of estrone, estradiol, and SHBG remained steady.

DHEA supplementation will generally increase levels of DHEA in the blood as well as serum androstenedione and testosterone. In one study, twenty-five milligrams of DHEA taken orally each day for one year led to higher serum DHEAS levels and higher levels of testosterone in a young man suffering from hypogonadism (severely low functioning testes). Overall, DHEA supplementation increases androgen levels in peripheral tissues, increases serum androstenedione, and improves functioning in most organ systems of the body. The majority of chronic diseases associated with male aging can be significantly helped with DHEA supplementation.

DHEA use has been shown to be associated with higher levels of energy and well-being, lower obesity and waist-to-hip ratios, enhanced libido and erectile ability, reduced depression, enhanced cognition, reduced death from coronary heart disease, and improved insulin sensitivity and glucose tolerance.

Suggested Dosage: The average dose is fifty milligrams per day. For men over fifty, this dose will usually raise blood levels of DHEA within two weeks to the same levels they experienced in their early twenties. Some people have taken dosages as high as 1,600 milligrams per day for extended periods. Side effects even at this high a dosage level are extremely rare.

When buying DHEA, make sure you are purchasing pharmaceutical-grade DHEA that is at least 98 percent pure. There is animal grade (70 percent pure) and food grade (95 percent pure). DHEA is readily available.

Side Effects: Some clinicians feel DHEA can exacerbate the mania stage of manic-depression, others feel it is contraindicated for men whose prostate-specific antigen (PSA) level is high (an indication of prostate disease). The only literature-noted side effect is masculinization (facial hair, etc.) in some women and the case of one woman who developed jaundice and liver problems after one week of use. It is not known if the latter side effect was related to the use of DHEA. Women seem most at risk of side effects.

Zinc

Zinc has significant effects on male sexuality, including sperm motility and production, erections, and even testosterone levels. Because the transformation of androstenedione to testosterone depends on a zinc-dependant enzyme, zinc intake significantly affects testosterone levels in the body. One study found that sixty milligrams of zinc daily for fifty days increased serum testosterone levels. Because DHT is metabolized from testosterone, a subsequent rise in DHT levels was also seen. Testosterone and DHT levels *only* increased in those men whose testosterone levels were low. Normal men experienced no increase.

Suggested Dosage: Twenty to forty milligrams per day for men over 40.

Side effects: Over time, zinc intake can cause copper depletion in the body. To counteract this, most zinc supplements come with copper added. At very high doses, zinc can cause nausea and upset stomach, skin rashes, depression, folate deficiency, and lower tolerance to alcohol.

Vitamin B$_5$ (Pantothenic acid)

Vitamin B$_5$ deficiency shows as adrenal atrophy accompanied by fatigue, headache, sleep irregularity, nausea, and abdominal problems. The vitamin is used by the body to keep the adrenal glands healthy and is often low in people suffering from exhausted or overworked adrenals. Men with low levels of androgens often have poorly functioning adrenal glands. Vitamin B$_5$ will support healthy adrenal function and the adrenal production of androgens.

Suggested Dosage: One hundred to five hundred milligrams daily.

Androstenedione (Andro)

Androstenedione, often called andro, is one of two androgens in the body that is converted directly into testosterone, making it a metabolic precursor of testosterone. The body converts DHEA to andro and then turns it (usually) into testosterone and (sometimes) into estrone, an estrogen. Andro and testosterone convert back and forth between each other using a specific zinc-dependant enzyme, 17-beta-hydroxysteroid dehydrogenase. Androstenedione is also sometimes made through an entirely different process in the body. Instead of the pathway: pregnenolone → 17a-hydroxypregnenolone → DHEA → andro, it is made: pregnenolone → progesterone → 17a-hydroxyprogesterone → andro. For this second pathway, the enzyme 17,20-lyase is used. Anything that reduces the levels of the particular enzyme (or the zinc it needs) that converts andro to testosterone, or that makes andro in the first place, results in lower levels of testosterone. Licorice, as noted in chapter 7, inhibits the 17,20-lyase enzyme and does reduce both serum testosterone and androstenedione. Interestingly, echinacea *(Echinacea purpurea)* has been found to *increase* levels of 17-hydroxysteroids in the body and has shown activity in the kidneys and adrenal glands as a 17-hydroxysteroid stimulant.

Androstenedione, compared with testosterone, is a weak androgen. Its importance for men is that it has been shown to increase testosterone levels when taken as a supplement. German researchers have found that a fifty-milligram dose of androstenedione can raise testosterone levels in normal men from 140 to 183 percent above normal. An East German study showed increased testosterone levels of up to 250 percent. However, the peak only lasts a few minutes, and testosterone levels slowly drop to baseline in a few hours. A more recent study by a California urologist found that after taking androstenedione, men experienced a rapid rise in testosterone levels of from 22 to 56 percent within ninety minutes. A placebo-controlled trial in 1997 showed that, compared to placebo, only those taking andro experienced increases of testosterone, about a twenty-four percent increase on average.

Men who take andro as a supplement commonly report feelings of increased well-being, energy, and strength. Because it causes a predictable peak in testosterone levels, some men take it ninety minutes prior to sex to stimulate sexual arousal and response or prior to exercise to get maximum effect from a workout.

Testosterone tends to peak in the body in midmorning, midafternoon, and between three and five a.m. As men age, the height of these peaks lowers, sometimes considerably and especially in those who are testosterone compromised. Some people have recommended that andro be taken upon rising, again at noon, and again before bed to simulate the body's normal patterns.

Suggested Dosage: Between fifty and one hundred milligrams three times per day. Some people preferred to allow the pill to dissolve under the tongue so that it entered the bloodstream directly instead of going through the liver and digestive system. Some research has indicated this was more effective. The androstenedione in pine pollen does in fact enter the blood directly when taken as a tincture. **Note:** Androstenedione as an

individual supplement is no longer legal. After the passage of the Anabolic Steroid Control Act in 2005, it has been considered a controlled
substance, despite the fact that since 1996 an estimated fifty million doses
of androstenedione have been taken with no reported side effects.

Dihydrotestosterone (DHT)

There is a growing controversy about DHT, its presence in the male body,
and what it does as men age. There is considerable controversy about
whether it should be used as a supplement, even with a prescription.

DHT is made from testosterone through the action of two enzymes—
Type I and Type II 5-alpha reductase. DHT is, in fact, much more powerful than testosterone. It binds ten times more powerfully to the body's
androgen receptors, it cannot be metabolized into estrogens (as can
testosterone), and it inhibits the action of aromatase (the enzyme that
converts testosterone to estradiol). DHT seems to act strongly to regulate the androgen/estrogen balance in the body. The controversy over
DHT arises because a number of people believe that it is responsible
for the current epidemic of prostate problems in men in the United
States. As a result, many people strongly advise that men not use DHT
supplementation and heavily support the use of pharmaceuticals that
interfere with the action of 5-alpha reductase to decrease DHT levels in
the body. There is growing evidence that these perspectives about DHT
are incorrect.

Some physicians, such as the French endocrinologist Bruno de Lig-
nieres, have suggested that the best treatment for an inflamed prostate
may, in fact, be DHT. His research has indicated that prostate problems
may be occurring not from the presence of DHT but from an imbalance
in the androgen/estrogen ratio. A growing body of research indicates
that estradiol levels are indeed a more likely initiator of prostate inflammation than DHT. Because DHT is not convertible to estradiol through
the action of aromatase, it could in fact help relieve prostate inflammation if this is correct. For more on this, see the section in chapter 8 on
benign prostatic hyperplasia (BPH) and prostatitis. A number of studies with DHT have borne this out. Research has shown *no* correlation

between DHT use and prostate enlargement in older men. Estradiol, but not DHT, has been found to act with SHBG to cause an eightfold increase in intracellular cyclic adenosine monophosphate (cAMP, a substance that increases cellular activity) in human BPH tissue, which causes increased growth of the prostate. Because DHT blocks binding of estradiol to SHBG, its presence completely negates the effects of estradiol. In fact, the use of DHT in clinical trials was found to lower levels of both estradiol and SHBG.

Clinical trials have also shown that during supplemental administration of DHT, men did not experience prostate enlargement and levels of serum PSA (prostate specific antigen—an indicator for prostate disease) did not increase, while urine stream strength did increase, showing that the prostate was shrinking. In other words, there *was* relief in the obstructive symptoms experienced by the patients who had BPH, not an increase, as there would be if DHT were the cause of prostate enlargement.

In human trials and clinical use, DHT has been found to increase androgen levels, aid feelings of well-being, counter many of the effects of low testosterone levels, and support better erections and libido. DHT topical gel containing seventy milligrams of DHT was found safe and effective when used in a three-month, double-blind, placebo-controlled, randomized clinical trial with thirty-three men over age sixty; all had low testosterone levels. The men experienced improved blood cholesterol levels, decreases in fat mass, and increases in muscle strength. The report notes that *"standard markers of prostate or cardiovascular diseases were not adversely affected by the DHT treatment"* (emphasis mine).

DHT is exceptionally important in the health of the body and there are growing reports that the widespread use of 5-alpha reductase inhibitors is having mild negative effects on muscle mass and even stronger negative impacts on normal male androgenization. DHT is in many ways the most important hormone in the development of male characteristics, not testosterone. Men who are born lacking the 5-alpha reductase enzyme develop little or no pubic hair, have an underdeveloped prostate and penis, and experience disrupted libido and sexual capacity. Weight lifters who take testosterone with 5-alpha reductase blockers have experienced reduced muscle enhancement in their muscle-building programs instead of more. DHT, it turns out, is crucial for the central nervous system and brain. It is vital in the organization and functioning of neural cells in the brain and has a greater neural impact than testosterone. Both testosterone and DHT increase the proliferation of androgen receptors in neural cells. However, testosterone's effects begin to fade after three hours, yet DHT maintains the increase for up to twenty-four hours. The brain converts the testosterone to estrogens when it needs estradiol to maintain healthy brain function, but it also converts testosterone to DHT through the use of 5-alpha reductase. The use of 5-alpha reductase blockers may, in fact, produce negative impacts on brain function because they are generic in their action, not specific to the prostate. DHT is also made in a number of peripheral target cells to carry out essential functions of the body. By blocking the action of 5-alpha reductase, pharmaceutical blockers prevent the brain and all other peripheral tissues from converting testosterone to DHT when they need it.

These new findings about DHT in the brain suggest that, as in the prostate, it is the correct balance of androgens to estrogen that create the healthiest functioning. Research has also begun to suggest that DHT and testosterone affect the body and specifically the prostate through very different mechanisms. Testosterone alone may be insufficient in keeping the body healthy, DHT is proving essential. In the rush to blame DHT as the culprit for an enlarged prostate, its general impacts on male health are being overlooked.

Suggested Dosage: Nearly the only place that DHT is available is in France where it is usually prescribed as a topical gel containing seventy milligrams.

Because of the controversy about DHT, you should educate yourself and decide whether you want to use it or not based on all available information. Bearing the controversy in mind, DHT is felt by many people to be contraindicated for men with prostatitis, BPH, and prostate cancer. It is definitely NOT for adolescent males, as it will interfere with normal hormonal development.

6 ANDROGENIC FOODS

Everybody, sooner or later, sits down to a banquet of consequences.

ROBERT LOUIS STEVENSON

There are a number of foods that have been found to possess androgenic actions and that can help restore androgen levels or the androgen/estrogen balance in men. They primarily work by supplying androgenic chemicals, stimulating androgenic hormone production in the body, or strengthening and toning the adrenal glands and kidneys. Another important factor, however, comes into play when looking at using foods to stimulate testosterone levels in the body. Scores of studies have found that one of the reliable indicators of low testosterone levels is having high BMI and waist circumference figures. BMI means body/mass index and is a measure of body fat based on height and weight. (The formula is: BMI = weight in kilograms divided by height in meters squared.) Research has found that the higher the BMI and the larger the waist circumference, the lower the testosterone. What this comes down to is the fatter you are, the lower your testosterone levels. This is because of the unique nature of fat cells, especially in the aging male.

Fat cells are not just storage sites for fat but are also a highly active endocrine system that produces a great many potent hormones. Among these are estrogens such as estradiol. Fat cells, especially around the waist, both store and produce estrogenic compounds. This is why the higher the BMI and waist circumference, the lower the testosterone levels.

The most important thing to do to raise testosterone levels naturally is to make sure that your body fat levels, especially around the waist, are not overly high. The easiest way to lower fat levels is to reduce fat intake in your meals for a few months or do a series of short juice fasts. Diet modification such as a ten-week, low-fat diet that is followed by a short three- to ten-day juice fast is the most efficient way to drop body fat. (A ten-week, low-fat diet is outlined in the Appendix.) Exercise, which is more useful for toning the muscles, is a very distant third. There is no need to be particularly fanatical about this; food nazis are some of the least fun people on the planet. I generally do a severely restricted diet or a fast of one sort or another every year, usually in the spring, usually for two or three weeks. Generally, I lose fifteen to twenty pounds, my energy levels, androgen levels, and immune function all increase. Then I eat how I want. The next spring, I am run down again and a bit overweight from being sedentary over the winter, so I do it again.

The kidneys and the small glands that sit atop them, the adrenal glands, are important in the production of androgens. Many of the herbs that enhance androgen production do so by affecting the kidneys, though more often it is the adrenal glands.

If your body fat levels are already moderately low or if you have done a low-fat diet to lower your BMI, the next thing to do is to increase the intake of foods that contain androgens or androgen-stimulating chemicals, and those that exert a tonic effect on the kidneys and adrenal glands. A number of plant foods do both.

THE KIDNEYS

The kidneys are tiny actually, only about four-and-a-half inches high, two to three inches wide, and an inch thick. But they filter some 190 quarts of water and scores of other substances out of the blood each day. (Though after age forty this begins decreasing about 10 percent per decade.) Most of these filtered substances are reabsorbed. Ninety-nine percent of the water is reabsorbed into the blood; only about three pints are excreted. Of the 270 grams of glucose (except in diabetes), all is reabsorbed, of the 1100 grams of chloride, only 10 grams are excreted; and of the 48 grams of urea, only 15 grams are excreted. The kidneys constantly monitor the amount of nitrogen, water, and electrolytic salts (sodium, potassium, and chloride) coming into the body and excrete just enough to keep the balance the same. They monitor the body's acid/alkali balance and through altering urine composition maintain the Ph of the body. To accomplish all this, the kidneys make and release enzymes and hormones that maintain the body's water, red blood cells, calcium, and phosphorous, the mineral content of the bones, and the diameter of capillaries, among other things. The adrenal glands that make so many important androgens for men sit just on top of the kidneys and are, in many respects, part of them.

The Kidneys' Enzymes and Hormones

The kidneys monitor the body's blood pressure constantly and raise and lower it through creating and releasing a hormone called renin, which the liver uses to make angiotensin. Renin also increases the size of that portion of the adrenal gland that produces aldosterone while angiotensin stimulates its production. (Aldosterone causes the kidneys to reabsorb more water and sodium.) Angiotensin also constricts the walls of arterioles, increases the strength of the heartbeat, and stimulates the pituitary gland to release antidiuretic hormone, which lowers the amount of water being excreted. These actions increase the blood pressure and intimately affect the levels of sodium and salt in the body.

The kidneys constantly monitor oxygen levels in the body's cells. When it is too low, they produce a hormone called erythropoietin, which stimulates the bone marrow to make and release more red blood cells. When oxygen levels return to optimum, the kidneys quit making erythropoietin. Through this process, the kidneys maintain the balance of red blood cells in the body.

The kidneys also make another hormone called calcitriol, a unique form of vitamin D. Vitamin D is in actuality not a vitamin but a type of steroidal hormone that is synthesized in a unique endocrine system in the body. During exposure to sunlight, the human skin converts a form of cholesterol to Vitamin D_3, the liver alters or metabolizes this again (into 25-hydroxycholcalciferol, aka 25-OHD3), and then the kidneys use that altered substance to make two highly biologically active hormones. One of them, calcitriol, acts on the cells of the intestine to increase absorption of calcium from the diet and direct it to the bones for bone formation. Calcitriol also regulates certain parathyroid hormones that maintain the body's levels of phosphorous. The kidneys constantly monitor the levels of calcium and phosphorous in the body and increase or decrease them as needed. Through calcitriol, the kidneys regulate bone mineralization and maintain the transfer of calcium to the bones to make them stronger. Thus they affect not only the bone marrow in the creation of red blood cells but also the bone itself.

Importantly, recent research has revealed that the kidneys also create enzymes that help to synthesize arginine. Arginine is an important precursor of nitric oxide (an erectile stimulant), stimulates sperm production and motility, boosts growth hormone release, and possesses wound-healing and immune-enhancing functions.

The kidneys also are highly responsive to steroidal hormones and possess a large number of estrogen receptor sites. Estrogens can bind to these sites in the kidneys, especially when estrogen levels in the body are high. This causes increases in body water levels, sodium content, and blood pressure.

Low androgen levels in men have an impact on kidney function. Research has shown that a healthy renin/angiotensin cycle is regulated by androgens through the action of a protein, the kidney androgen-regulated protein (Kap). This takes place in the part of the kidney that also produces the calcitriol that regulates bone mineralization and density. High estrogen/low androgen levels produce different actions than when these levels are normal, especially in this part of the kidneys. This possibly explains why men suffer from osteoporosis at much higher rates as they move into middle age and their androgen and testosterone levels change. It also explains to some extent the significant alteration for middle-aged men in how their bodies maintain water and sodium levels during sleep. Research has shown that healthy kidneys in men are highly dependant on testosterone and that men with kidney disease have far higher levels of estrogens in their bodies and much lower levels of testosterone. Estrogens, it is now known, also stimulate the production of epidermal growth factor in the kidneys, which testosterone does not do. This growth factor has been linked to some types of prostate cancer, and the estrogen-initiated production of epidermal growth factor in the kidneys is a potential contributing cause.

THE ADRENAL GLANDS

The adrenal glands, the two tiny pyramid-shaped organs that sit on top of the kidneys, are named for their location. *Ad* means near, *renal* is the Latin for kidney. The outer layer of the adrenal gland, the cortex, and the inner layer, the medulla, produce nearly 150 different essential hormones. The cortex itself produces more than two dozen important hormones, for example: cortisol, cortisone, aldosterone, DHEA, DHEAS, DHT, androstenedione, and testosterone. The adrenal medulla produces the most famous of the adrenal hormones, adrenaline (real name: epinephrine; adrenaline is actually the name of a synthetic drug), and its close relative noradrenaline (aka norepinephrine). The adrenal glands are responsible for nearly 50 percent of all the androgens in a man's body. They produce significant quantities of male hormones, 90 percent of the body's DHEA, powerful anti-inflammatories such as cortisol, and fright-flight-or-fight hormones like adrenaline. They are closely tied to the testes, heart, lungs, and kidneys through intricate biofeedback loops and hormonal exchange systems.

Actions of Adrenal Hormones

Stress has powerful impacts on this hormonal exchange system. Under continued stress, the body will release high, constant levels of stress hormones such as cortisol and epinephrine. Cortisol blocks inflammation, regulates the water content of blood, and modifies blood sugar levels by releasing glucose from fats and proteins when it is needed. It also interferes with the conversion of tryptophan to serotonin, which causes an increase in wakefulness. Over time, chronic high cortisol levels can cause insomnia and constant poor sleep. In early morning, cortisol levels are high, in the evening they are low.

Epinephrine is used by the body as a short-burst, high-alert response to danger. It stimulates heart action, increases the diameter of air passages to stimulate oxygen uptake, and speeds up the liver's glucose production. Constant stress results in high levels of both cortisol and epinephrine and such physical symptoms as increased metabolism, hyper-wakefulness, rapid heart beat, increased blood pressure, nervousness, increased stomach acid, increased muscle tension, and higher levels of emotional aggressiveness. Caffeine, especially at the levels found in coffee, stimulates the production of epinephrine and prevents its breakdown, which is why drinking coffee produces so many of the same symptoms.

Of significant importance is that as cortisol levels rise, DHEA levels decrease. The shift to cortisol metabolism inhibits DHEA production. This lowers the levels of androgens in the body. The adrenal glands can become exhausted or suffer overstimulation after years of high cortisol production. This is especially serious in men with decreased androgen levels. Once the adrenals become overtaxed or exhausted, energy levels decline both from lack of normal epinephrine/cortisol levels and low androgen levels.

THE KIDNEYS AND ADRENAL GLANDS IN CHINESE MEDICINE

While many of the actions of the kidney/adrenal system are new to Western science, they are not to the Chinese. Chinese physicians have long understood the close connection of the kidneys to the heart and intestines. Within their system, disharmony between the heart and kidney or kidney and intestines was known to be the cause of numerous diseases, including kidney stones, urinary gravel, and certain blood circulation problems. Chinese physicians also understood the connection of the kidney to low androgen levels. They call it "empty kidney-glands," meaning there is insufficient production of vital hormones. This is especially perceptive in that the term for this condition occurred many thousands of years before any Western scientist knew that the adrenals produce many of the essential hormones and androgens for male health. The kidneys are considered to be an organ of balance and do, within the Chinese system, affect the functioning of the inner ear. Vertigo (and even tinnitus) can be a sign of a disordered kidney, the imbalance in the kidney causing a literal inability to balance.

ANDROGENIC TONICS FOR THE ADRENAL GLANDS AND KIDNEYS

There is one primary herb for the kidney/adrenal system that also supplies androgens: celery. Its regular use as a juice has profound impacts on both androgen and energy levels. Common sweet corn also has strong impacts on the kidney/adrenal system.

As always, you should try to buy only organic vegetables and herbs. Not only will this avoid as much chemical contaminants as possible but the mineral and vitamin contents of organic foods are much higher. Over the past forty years, the mineral content of most vegetables has declined between 25 and 35 percent because of the way they are grown.

If you do suffer from adrenal exhaustion in particular and not just low androgen levels, you might try a daily regimen of juice made from one cup of corn kernels and three to four stalks of celery as well as two hundred milligrams of eleuthero, five hundred milligrams of nettle root, two hundred milligrams of vitamin B_5, and twenty milligrams of zinc for three to six months.

Celery (Apium graveolens)

Besides containing significant amounts of androgen-like chemicals, celery is exceptional for lowering blood pressure and helping the circulatory system and also has a number of things to recommend its use for the health of the kidneys and adrenals.

Two stalks of celery contain (approximately) the following nutrients: 275 milligrams potassium, 30 milligrams magnesium, 35 milligrams calcium, 20 milligrams phosphorous, 90 milligrams sodium, 225 international units (IU) vitamin A, 8 milligrams vitamin C, 0.2 milligrams iron,

8 micrograms folic acid, and trace amounts of thiamine, riboflavin, niacin, and vitamin B$_6$.

Celery is closely related to a number of very powerful medicinal plants: osha *(Ligusticum porterii)*, angelica *(Angelica archangelica)*, and lomatium *(Lomatium dissectum)*. It is not surprising, then, that celery also possesses a number of very powerful medicinal actions. Like these other plants, celery is antimicrobial, antibacterial, slightly antiviral, antispasmodic, and anti-inflamatory.

Celery is especially useful for lowering blood pressure. It contains a compound called 3-n-butyl phthalide that can lower blood pressure about fourteen percent when taken in sufficient quantities. It is also high in apigenin, a blood-vessel dilator that also helps lower blood pressure. Eating three to four celery stalks will supply the necessary amount of both compounds to lower blood pressure. Celery also contains a large number of compounds that act like calcium-channel blockers and that help reduce and prevent angina. The apigenin, magnesium, potassium, and another compound, apiin in celery, make it a useful herb for cardiac arrhythmia, as well. In a number of studies, celery juice has also been found to significantly reduce cholesterol levels in the blood. Celery is a strong antioxidant and is also reliably effective in lowering the levels of uric acid in the body by stimulating its excretion in the urine. Historically, this has made celery a primary remedy for gout. Normally the seeds are used, but the fresh juice, while slightly weaker in action, produces the same result. Celery has also been found effective for helping alleviate arthritis and rheumatic complaints, skin rashes and diseases, nervousness (especially when accompanied by anxiety), upset stomach and digestive system, and gallstones.

But celery's major areas of importance are its impacts on the kidneys. Its wide-ranging impacts on kidney function help the removal of toxins from the body through the kidneys by enhancing kidney function and urine flow. Because part of the primary function of the kidneys is to filter the blood and maintain the body's electrolyte balance, the regular ingestion of celery juice supports optimum filtration and electrolyte balances. Electrolyte balance is also enhanced because of the large amounts of primary electrolytes in celery, including calcium, magnesium, and potassium.

Celery is a specific remedy for the kidneys. It is a kidney tonic, an antimicrobial, antispasmodic, and anti-inflammatory for the urinary passage, reduces kidney stone formation, increases urine flow (a diuretic), and (in Chinese medicine) helps alleviate dizziness. Celery's volatile oil, apiol, is excreted through the urinary tract and acts as a mild, but reliable urinary system antiseptic.

Researchers have also found a male steroid in celery. The chemical, 5 alpha-androst-16-en-3 alpha-ol, and its related 3-ketone combine to form the chemicals that a number of animals use to stimulate sexual arousal in the female; they are a sign of elevated sexual hormones in the male and its readiness to mate. The two compounds are closely related in structure to both androstenedione and testosterone. They are present in celery at about the level of eight nanograms per gram of fresh celery, a moderately high level. This perhaps explains why celery has long been used as a sexual tonic for men. **Note:** Parsnip *(Pastinaca sativa)* also contains these same androgenic chemicals and can be added to the diet regularly to help enhance androgen levels.

Of further importance to enhancing testosterone levels and the health of the male reproductive system recent research on apigenin has found it to have a much greater range of action than merely acting as a blood-vessel dilator. Apigenin has been shown to suppress androgen-independent prostatic tumor cells and also acts as a fairly strong aromatase inhibitor. In numerous studies it has been found to significantly inhibit the conversion of testosterone to estradiol.

In short, celery affects the entire urinary network, much of the reproductive system, and most of the bodily systems that the kidneys affect: heart, digestive system, adrenal glands, and blood vessels.

Suggested Dosage: Three to four celery stalks juiced daily makes three to four ounces of juice. Best as an androgen/kidney tonic if blended with corn (see next listing).

For Urinary Tract Infections: Celery *seed,* like many seeds of medicinal plants, is stronger in some of the medicinal actions of celery, especially for urinary tract infections. (It is also good for arthritis, gout, and kidney stones.) If you have a urinary tract infection, you may want to add a squirt of celery seed tincture to your juice each morning as well. The tincture is usually available at health food stores.

Side Effects: Fresh celery juice, taken in quantity, will cause a slight numbing to the tongue. Large doses of celery juice are contraindicated in kidney disease. The roots will sometimes, because of improper storage, become infected with yeasts that can raise the content of a substance called furocumarin in the roots by as much as 200 percent. These furocumarin-enhanced roots can cause phototoxicosis (skin sensitivity to light). Use only fresh celery. In rare circumstances, celery can cause allergic reactions in some individuals to the severity of anaphylactic shock. Do not use if you have a history of allergic reaction to celery or similar plants.

Corn (Zea mays)

Although most people do not realize it, corn is a specific tonic for the whole urinary tract, including the adrenal glands. The corn kernels, corn silk, and the pollen are all kidney/adrenal specific, though the pollen is somewhat difficult to find.

Corn silk is highly effective for cystitis, acute and chronic inflammations of the bladder, urethritis, and prostatitis. Corn pollen has been used similarly to pine pollen in a number of cultures as a restorative of male vitality, and contains many of the same amino acids and vitamins that are found in pine pollen. Corn pollen is part of the medicinal blend Cernilton, the rye grass pollen mixture that is so successful in treating prostate disease. And importantly, in cases of androgen deficiency, corn juice stimulates the production and release of luteinizing hormone (LH). This hormone binds to sites on the Leydig cells in the testes, which stimulates the synthesis and secretion of testosterone. In a number of studies, corn was found to increase the levels of androgens in test animals.

Corn is an anodyne (soothing pain), a diuretic (increasing urine expression), demulcent (soothing to mucous membranes), anti-inflammatory, anti-spasmodic, and tonic. The Spanish writer Garcilaso de la Vega (1539–1616) commented that he was highly impressed:

. . . with the remarkable curative properties of corn, which is not only the principle article of food in America, but is also of benefit in the treatment of the kidneys and bladder, among which are calculus and retention of urine. And the best proof I can give of this is that the Indians, whose usual drink is made of corn, are afflicted with none of these diseases.[1]

While most people don't think of drinking corn, it has been used for some ten thousand years to make chicha, a kind of beer unique to the Americas. While chicha is difficult to find in the northern hemisphere, you can easily run corn kernels through a juicer each morning to obtain the juice. As the corn juice is a bit thick, I blend it with four ounces of celery juice, a really delicious combination. There is no better overall tonic for the kidney/adrenal system than this combination.

Suggested Dosage: Two to four ounces juiced organic corn kernels daily (about 2–4 ounces of kernels).

Corn Silk: Corn silk is most often used for inflammation in the urinary tract. In a number of clinical trials, it has been found to be especially effective in reducing excess water retention, swelling, and edema—all problems that occur from estrogen excess. The stigmas—the four- to eight-inch-long fine, silky threads that you pull off corn on the cob as you shuck it—are what is normally used for urinary tract problems. They are best used fresh. A tea or tincture made from corn silk can be added to the juice daily if you are experiencing specific urinary tract problems.

Corn Silk Suggested Dosage: Steep two teaspoons of the silk in eight ounces of hot water for fifteen minutes and drink the tea three times per day. The tincture may be purchased in health food stores: take three to six milliliters (¾–1½ tsp.) of the tincture three times daily.

Androgen/Adrenal Green Drink: I find the best way to use celery and corn for androgen increase and supporting kidney/adrenal health is as a fresh juice. They go into the system much more quickly, and the impact is much stronger. I usually drink it on an empty stomach each morning.

Here is a recipe for androgen/adrenal green drink that I have used for a long time. It also contains cucumber, kale, spinach, and radish.

Androgen/Adrenal Green Drink

2 stalks fresh celery

1 cup corn kernels

½ cucumber

1 large fresh kale leaf

½ cup fresh spinach

(optional: 1–3 radishes)

Juice all the vegetables in a juicer.

Cucumber (Cucumis sativus)

One-half an average cucumber contains 260 IU vitamin A, 220 milligrams potassium, 20 micrograms folic acid, 20 milligrams calcium, 15 milligrams magnesium, 25 milligrams phosphorous, 5 milligrams sodium, moderate amounts of silica and chlorophyll, and trace amounts of vitamin C, thiamine, riboflavin, niacin, vitamin B_6, boron, and iron.

Cucumbers are a mild diuretic; their seeds possess mild tonic actions on the kidneys, help prevent kidney stones, and promote uric acid excretion from the body. Cucumbers, especially the peels, are exceptionally good for promoting healthy skin, keeping it elastic, and reducing wrinkles. I like their addition to green drinks because they contribute a LOT of water, diluting the intensity of the other plants in the mixture.

Suggested Dosage: One-half cucumber per green drink. Do not peel cucumbers, juice them whole.

Kale (Brassica oleracea)

Kale is especially high in beneficial nutrients such as carotenes and chlorophyll. One large kale leaf with stem (about 3 ounces) contains 10,000 IU vitamin A, 100 milligrams vitamin C, 175 micrograms folic acid, 250 milligrams potassium, 200 milligrams calcium, 2 milligrams iron, 15 milligrams magnesium, 60 milligrams phosphorous, 3 milligrams sodium, 2 milligrams niacin, and trace amounts of thiamine, riboflavin, vitamin B_6, copper, manganese, and zinc.

A cup of kale or collard greens has more calcium than a glass of milk and, in this form (juiced), is much better assimilated into the body. Kale, like other members of the *Brassica* family such as cabbage, broccoli, and cauliflower, possesses potent anticancer compounds and a rich supply of antioxidants.

Suggested Dosage: One large leaf with stem per green drink.

Spinach (Spinacia oleracea)

Like other dark green leafy vegetables, spinach contains large amounts of chlorophyll and carotenes—both of which offer potent protection against cancer. One cup of fresh, raw spinach contains 3750 IU vitamin A, 16 milligrams vitamin C, 110 micrograms folic acid, 300 milligrams potassium, 60 milligrams calcium, 1.5 milligrams iron, 45 milligrams magnesium, 30 milligrams phosphorous, 22 milligrams sodium, and trace amounts of thiamine, riboflavin, niacin, and vitamin B_6.

Suggested Dosage: ½ cup of fresh spinach.

Radish (Raphanus sativus)

There are a number of different types of radishes; all can be used and are of benefit. The most commonly known is the red radish, but there is a Japanese radish, the daikon, that looks something like a white carrot. There are also black radishes, which are used mostly in Russia and the Eastern European countries. They look much like a very black beet, although inside they possess the normal crisp, white flesh of a radish. All three taste much the same. Daikon radishes are always available in oriental markets and sometimes in health food stores. Black radishes can mostly be found in neighborhood markets that have large numbers of Russian or Polish customers.

A single medium-sized red radish contains in the neighborhood of 25 milligrams potassium, 2.5 milligrams each of calcium and phosphorous, 1.5 milligrams of sodium, 1 IU of vitamin A, 2 milligrams of vitamin C, and varying traces of magnesium, selenium, iron and zinc.

Radishes tend to normalize the production of thyroxine in the thyroid gland. If too much T4 is being produced radishes bring levels up, if too little, they lower them. They are, in fact, a thyroid tonic herb and can be very helpful in treating thyroid problems. Radishes contain a unique compound, raphinin, that normalizes not only thyroxine but also calcitonin, another hormone produced in the thyroid gland. Thyroid-produced calcitonin controls the amount of calcium released into the blood and affects the amount of calcium laid down in the bones during bone matrix formation. With regular intake of radishes or radish juice the thyroid production of these compounds is normalized. Russian physicians have successfully used radishes for decades for alleviating both hyperthyroidism and hypothyroidism.

Radishes have been found in a number of clinical studies in Malaysia to be powerful inhibitors of kidney stones in prior sufferers who consume them regularly. They also help the liver work with fat intake in the diet more effectively, seem to help break up fat deposits in fatty liver conditions, and help break up gallstones in the gallbladder.

Suggested Dosage: One to three medium-sized red radishes, juiced, or the equivalent amount of juiced daikon or black radish, daily. They are spicy, as you know, so start with one and then use more if you like it.

OTHER ANDROGENIC FOODS

There are a few other androgenic foods that are helpful in increasing androgen levels: oats, garlic, pine nuts, and red meat.

Oats (Avena sativa)

Green oats (basically the fresh green oatmeal plant in seed) have been found to increase testosterone levels in men in at least one study; various other studies support this androgenic activity. In vivo research has found that oats, dried and added to animal diets, increase the release of luteinizing hormone (LH), which stimulates the creation and release of testosterone into the bloodstream. Oats were official as a sexual tonic and stimulant in older German pharmacopoeias and are listed as a common doctor-prescribed unofficial herb for this use in the current German Commission E Monographs on herbal medicine.

Oats also contain a number of alkaloids, including trigonelline and avenine, that have central nervous system relaxant activity and which help relax the people who eat them regularly. This relaxant activity makes oats one of the best long-term foods for stressed nerves, tension, nervous debility, and exhaustion. This kind of stress reduction in many instances helps male sexual function.

Oats are also high in Vitamin E, which is an essential vitamin for sexual health as it helps prevent atherosclerosis and prostate disease. Oatmeal also contains about 70 percent fiber and is very high in polyunsaturated fatty acids. Both these factors contribute greatly to lowering cholesterol levels in the blood and rectifying or preventing atherosclerosis (fat clogging the arteries and veins), one of the major factors affecting erectile function.

Oats are best used long term, the effects build up over time and increase in effectiveness the longer oats are eaten. In general, effects begin to be noticed after three months and increase throughout the first year.

Suggested Dosage: Eat one bowl of oatmeal per day.

Garlic (Allium sativum)

Garlic, a member of the lily family, has a long history as a sexual tonic for men. After ginseng, it is perhaps one of the most intensely studied medicinal plants on Earth. There have been a substantial number of clinical trials, including double-blind, placebo-controlled, crossover studies. Garlic has shown consistent activity in increasing testosterone levels, stimulating the production of sperm, increasing sexual desire, reducing atherosclerosis, and alleviating cardiac arrhythmia, diabetes, hypertension, and the effects of a depressed immune system.

Suggested Dosage: Garlic and its close relative, onion, which has many of the same properties, should be liberally added to the diet. Garlic supplements can also be used. Follow the directions on the bottle.

Herb/Drug Interactions: Avoid garlic if you are taking anticoagulants, paracetamol (acetaminophen), or chlorpropamide.

Red Meat

Regular consumption of red meat, one to three times per week, is important for keeping androgen levels high. Studies have shown that reducing the intake of meat and the dietary fats from meats reduces serum androgen levels in men. In one study, thirty healthy men had their diets changed to reduce their meat intake and lower their ratio of polyunsaturated fats to saturated fatty acids. After six weeks, their levels of total serum testosterone, androstenedione, and free testosterone declined an average of 10 percent.

Suggested Dosage: Organic or wild, red meat once per week.

Pine Nuts *(Pinus semen)*

Pine nuts have been used in every ecoregion, and they occur as both a nutritional and aphrodisiacal food. They can be made into soups, ground into flour for breads, eaten raw, roasted, and added to dishes like pesto.

For thousands of years and among such different cultures as the Romans, Greeks, Arabians, and Asians, pine nuts have been considered an aphrodisiac. The Greek physician Galen suggested that a mixture of honey, almonds, and pine nuts, eaten on three consecutive evenings, would produce an increase in male vitality. Also, Ovid, the Roman poet, provides a list of aphrodisiacs in his *Ars Amatoria* (The Art of Love), which includes "the nuts that the sharp-leaved pine brings forth." There is good reason for this long-standing recognition that pine nuts can increase male vitality.

Like pine pollen, pine nuts also contain testosterone, and they are also highly nutritious. Although the nutrients in pine nuts vary between species, a good indication of their nutritional power can be seen from a look at the nut of the American pinyon pine. One ounce of pinion nuts contains 161 calories and 3.3 grams of protein, 5.5 grams of carbohydrates, 2.7 grams of saturated fat, 6.5 grams of monounsaturated fat, 7.28 grams of polyunsaturated fat, 2.3 milligrams of calcium, 10 milligrams of phosphorous, 20 milligrams of sodium, 178 milligrams of potassium, 0.88 milligrams of iron, 8.2 IU of vitamin A, 0.35 milligrams of thiamin, 0.05 milligrams of riboflavin, and 1 milligram of niacin. As an example of how nuts from different pines can vary, Spanish pine nuts (pignolias) contain nearly 7 grams of protein and 144 milligrams of phosphorous but only 1 milligram of sodium, with the other constituents being about identical with those of pinyon pine nuts. All pine nuts are high in omega-3 oils and amino acids such as arginine.

The green cones are picked by hand from autumn to spring and piled to dry. As they dry, the cones open and allow the hull-covered seeds, called pine nuts, to be extracted by either mechanical or hand thrashing. They are then further dried, and the nuts hulled by milling. The primary species used (in order) are *P. pinea, P. koraiensis,* and *P. edulis* (the pinyon pine), while at least ten others are used for food around the world. Unfortunately, it is often impossible to find out which species you are buying because few nut suppliers list the tree species on their packages. Sometimes, to make it even more difficult, the different species are intermingled for sale. (Some Internet companies do say which species they sell.) Pine nuts can go rancid, so they should be used moderately quickly; unrefrigerated, they last three months, refrigerated, six months. Pine nuts are readily available on the Internet from nut companies and in many stores, especially during the fall harvesting season.

Suggested Dosage: Eat as much and as often as desired.

Side Effects: Nut sensitivities. Pine nuts also contain the female hormones estrone and estradiol. To date, I have been unable to find the exact levels. Anecdotal evidence indicates that, at least in this instance, their presence is not usually a problem affecting male androgen levels.

7 TESTOSTERONE ANTAGONISTS
Things to Avoid

Hops is not much use for a human being, since it causes his melancholy to increase, gives him a sad mind, and makes his intestines heavy.

HILDEGARD OF BINGEN, 1159 CE

Just as there are substances that increase androgen levels and androgenic activity in men, there are also substances that can significantly lower or suppress them. If you are having trouble with your levels of testosterone or your androgen/estrogen ratio, you should especially avoid consuming any quantity of licorice, black cohosh, and hops. Each of these plants contains substances that are either potent estrogens, act as androgen antagonists, or interfere with the conversion of prohormones into androgens, or stimulate the conversion of androgens into estrogens.

Licorice (Glycyrrhiza glabra)

Licorice is an exceptionally good herb for a great many things, however, it should be used sparingly, if at all, and only for conditions for which nothing else will do. Licorice has highly negative effects on men's androgen levels and hormonal functioning. In numerous human studies, for example, it has been found to inhibit the actions of 11-beta-hydroxysteroid dehydrogenase, which is used to convert cortisol to cortisone and back again as each compound is needed. Cortisol is highly active in the body, and a specific ratio is naturally maintained between cortisol and cortisone in order to minimize the negative effects of cortisol. (Natural cortisone is structurally different than pharmaceutical cortisone preparations. The body converts both types of cortisone to cortisol to make them active.) By inhibiting 11-beta-hydroxysteroid dehydrogenase, licorice upsets the cortisol/cortisone ratio. Any imbalance in this ratio will usually have strongly negative side effects.

High cortisol levels have been linked to impaired immune health, reduced ability to utilize glucose in the blood, increased bone loss, osteoporosis, increased fat accumulation around the hips and waist, impaired memory and learning, destruction of brain cells, and impaired skin growth and regeneration. Cortisol levels sometimes rise in the bodies of weight lifters who are training intensively. In such cases, it will cause the breakdown of muscle tissue because cortisol converts proteins in the muscles into glucose as a source of energy. High cortisol levels also cause a lowering of testosterone levels in the body; basically, cortisol appears to suppress testosterone. Part of the reason for this is that the steroid hormone pregnenolone is converted to cortisol through enzymatic activity. If it is not converted to cortisol, pregnenolone is instead turned into testosterone and other DHEA-based androgens. The shifting of the body to cortisol production tends to lower DHEA production and, as a result, testosterone levels.

In addition, licorice actually restricts the conversion of 17-hydroxy-progesterone into the androgen androstenedione (which itself becomes testosterone and DHT) by inhibiting the 17,20-lyase enzyme. Clinical studies have found that the use of licorice by men decreases levels of both serum testosterone and androstenedione while raising levels of progesterone. This directly results in decreased libido and various forms of sexual dysfunction. To compound this dynamic, licorice also contains at least seven estrogenic compounds. Two of them are direct estrogens (rather than estrogen mimics): clycestrone and estriol. Clycestrone is similar to estrone but is only $\frac{1}{533}$ as potent. Estriol is (as is estrogen) one of the three primary estrogenic steroids produced in the body. Usually, high levels of estriol are present only in women during pregnancy.

To sum up, licorice intake increases cortisol levels in the body, lowers the production of testosterone, and directly increases levels of estrogens. It also possesses a number of other, sometimes serious, side effects from continued use or the use of high levels of the extracts.

Because of these cumulative impacts, men who are concerned about the androgen/estrogen ratio in their bodies should not use licorice except short term for specific conditions such as stomach ulcers. Although most people do not know it, licorice is used with some frequency in dark beers to increase head, as a coloring agent, and to sweeten the end product (see Hops listing below).

Black Cohosh (Cimicifuga racesmosa)

Black cohosh is highly estrogenic and is often used for normalizing female hormonal levels during menopause and to alleviate menopausal symptoms such as hot flashes. It has shown an antagonist activity toward the production and release of luteinizing hormone (LH), which is essential in testosterone production. It is sometimes used by men for muscle pain as it is an exceptionally good antispasmodic. It should be avoided by men with androgenic imbalances unless no other herb will do.

Hops (Humulus lupulus)

Hops is best known for its use in beer. The majority of physicians and men overlook its potent chemicals and do not realize that beer itself can significantly alter male androgen levels. German beer makers noticed long ago that the young women who picked hops in the fields commonly experienced early menstrual periods. Eventually, researchers discovered the reason—hops is perhaps one of the most powerfully estrogenic plants on Earth. Just 100 grams of hops (about 3.5 ounces) contains anywhere from thirty thousand to three hundred thousand IUs of estrogens, depending on the type of hops. Most of it is the very potent estrogen estradiol. Estradiol, as it is taken into the male body, causes a direct lowering of testosterone levels in the testes and an increase in SHBG levels, which then binds up even more free testosterone in the bloodstream.

The estradiol in hops has also been found to directly interfere with the ability of the testes Leydig cells to produce testosterone. The presence of this highly estrogenic substance in beer is not an accident.

Prior to the German Beer Purity Act of 1516, beer almost never contained hops. In fact, more than one hundred different plants were used in brewing beer for at least ten thousand years prior to the introduction of hops in the middle ages. For the last thousand years of that period, the most dominant form of "beer" was called gruit, which contained a mixture of yarrow, bog myrtle, and marsh rosemary. These herbs, especially in beer, are sexually and mentally stimulating. (It is rare to become sleepy when drinking un-hopped beers.) The Catholic Church had a monopoly on the production of gruit, but competing merchants and the Protestants worked together to break that monopoly and force the removal of all sexually stimulating herbs from beer. They replaced them with an herb that puts the drinker to sleep and dulls sexual drive in the male. The legislative arguments of the day all hinged on the issue of the stimulating effects of other herbs that were used in beer. A pilsner, for example, was originally a henbane beer (*pilsen* means "henbane"), which is an incredibly strong, psychoactive beer, used earlier in history by German berserkers before battle. The German Beer Purity Act was, in effect, the first drug control law ever enacted.

Beer, so highly touted as sexy in television commercials, in actuality can powerfully inhibit sexual strength in men. There is a well-known condition in England—Brewer's Droop—that occurs from middle-aged brewers' extensive handling of hops plants. The plant chemistries readily transmit through the men's skin just as they did in the young women in the fields. Very few physicians have looked at any correlation between beer drinking and androgen levels or erectile dysfunction problems in their patients. (How many men on Viagra are heavy beer drinkers?) However, the physician Eugene Shippen in *The Testosterone Syndrome* comments that one of his patients, undergoing pharmaceutical testosterone replacement therapy, showed no response to the testosterone *until he reduced his beer intake to one to two beers a night from six to seven.*[1] Hops is extremely potent and *its consumption should be limited if not completely excluded during all androgen replacement therapy.* These effects can be exacerbated if the beers you buy also contain licorice (see Licorice section at beginning of chapter), a fact that will not be noted on the beer label.

It is possible to buy beer that does not interfere with androgen levels, although it can be somewhat hard to find. Some microbreweries and brew pubs are now making traditional gruits. Check the brew pubs in your town. However, the best source is Bruce Williams, a Scottish brewer who is bringing back the traditional ales of Europe and especially Scotland (i.e., pre-hopped European beers). He has five in production, and they can often be found in larger American cities at any store that carries a wide selection of unusual beers. The heather ale is excellent but perhaps more useful would be the traditional pine ale made from the Scotch pine, *Pinus sylvestris,* whose pollen contains testosterone.

It is also best to buy beers that are bottle-conditioned. Bottle-conditioned beers are carbonated in the bottle and as such contain live yeasts. These yeasts (most commonly *Saccharomyces cerevisiae*) are highly nutritive. They are extremely high in protein, glucose tolerance factor, and B vitamins—especially niacin and B_1. Glucose tolerance factor, because it helps regulate blood sugar levels, can help with many of the problems associated with diabetes. Brewer's yeast contains the highest levels of glucose tolerance factor of any food. It has also been found to reduce serum cholesterol and triglyceride levels and newer research has indicated that *S. cerevisiae* yeasts may have direct enhancement impacts on androgen activity in the body.

And since I am on the subject . . .

ALCOHOL AND MALE HEALTH

The United States is undergoing one of its periodic bouts of puritanitis (a spasming or inflammation of the Puritan Reflex). In spite of this, alcohol has been with the human species a long time. It is a *naturally* occurring substance, found throughout nature, and many living organisms are known to imbibe—the birds *and* the bees. Life, in fact, could not exist without the fermentation that both bacteria and yeasts provide. Nearly all indigenous cultures on Earth ferment and have done so for between ten thousand and thirty thousand years. Beer anthropologists (yes, they exist) have found significant evidence that the Egyptians settled where they did and developed agriculture and cities because they discovered that the naturally growing grain in that region could be fermented. In other words, civilization began when we started *drinking,* not when we starting thinking.

Alcohol is exceptionally good for the body *in moderation.* It stimulates the functioning of most organs, especially the liver and brain, to more optimum levels of health. However, in large quantities, alcohol's well-known negative effects come into play. Overuse leads to highly adverse effects on, not surprisingly, the liver and brain; basically, a case of overstimulation. Still, it is important to note that alcohol consumption significantly increases the metabolic conversion of androgenic precursors to more potent androgens (basically DHEA to androstenediol). Moderate alcohol consumption has also been found to increase the production of androgens by the adrenal glands and to promote healthy androgen levels in the body. However, ingesting large quantities of alcohol can exhaust the body's androgen levels and even interfere with their production. In rats, high alcohol intake over short time spans causes the leeching of all DHEA from the brain. While in humans, sustained high levels of alcohol have been found to reduce levels of testosterone and other androgens. Consistently high levels of alcohol cause the accumulation of tetrahydroisoquinoline alkaloids, which inhibit production of testosterone by Leydig cells in the testes. Tetrahydroisoquinoline alkaloids have been found to be as potent in that respect as the female hormone estradiol. They also interfere with the liver's ability to remove estrogen from the body by interfering with the liver's cytochrome P-450 system (the part of the liver concerned with estrogen removal).

Naturally occurring fermentations have been shown to be much healthier for the human body—that is, wines and bottle-conditioned beers, especially beers that do not contain hops. Most studies have shown that one to two drinks of alcohol per day are associated with higher levels of health. More than that and the level of health may begin to decline. Grapes also possess anti-aromatase activity (helping in preventing the conversion of testosterone to estradiol) and antioxidant properties (keeping cellular vitality high). Red wines also contain polyphenols, which are exceptionally good at regulating the impacts of fat on the health of the body. Alcohol content is normally limited to around 12 percent in nature—levels higher than that kill the yeast. It is primarily when alcohol content is concentrated beyond that level (as with distilled drinks), when the yeasts are removed (they counteract many of the side effects of alcohol ingestion, such as the loss of B vitamins), or when it is consumed to excess (as we do with sugar or fat) that side effects begin to be seen.

Grapefruit (*Citrus paradisi*)

I am pleased to finally find a good reason for my long dislike of grapefruit. Through a number of avenues (especially impacts on the cytochrome P450 system that breaks down estrogens in the liver), grapefruit interferes with the removal of estrogens from the body, increasing overall estrogen levels. It should be avoided by men following an androgen enhancement protocol . . . well, probably by all men.

OTHER THINGS TO AVOID

There are a number of substances that interfere with the removal of estrogen from the male body. (In essence, they increase estrogen levels by inhibiting the P450 phase I enzyme in the liver that breaks down estrogen.) If you are struggling with an impaired androgen/estrogen ratio, it is important to understand that these substances can have a strong impact on estrogen levels.

- Anti-inflammatories: ibuprofen, ketoprofen, diclofenac, acetaminophen, aspirin, propoxyphene.
- Antibiotics: sulfa drugs, tetracyclines, penicillins, cefazolins, erythromycins, floxins, isoniazid.
- Antifungals: miconazole, itraconazole, fluconazole, ketoconazole.

- Statins (cholesterol-lowering drugs): lovastatin, simvistatin.
- Antidepressants: fluoxetine, fluvoxamine, paroxetine, sertraline.
- Antipsychotics: chlorpromazine, haloperidol.
- Heart/Blood Pressure Medications: propranolol, quinidine, amiodarone (this also inhibits testosterone production), warfarin, methyldopa.
- Calcium Channel Blockers: antacids, omeprazole, cimetidine.

8 ENHANCING MALE SEXUALITY
Erectile Strength, Sperm Production and Motility, and Prostate Health

*The number of sperm cells released in a single
ejaculation of one man is 175 thousand times more
than the number of eggs a woman produces in her
entire lifetime. It can be more than the number of
people in North America; hundreds of millions.*

LYN MARGULIS AND DORIAN SAGAN,

MYSTERY DANCE

William Masters and Virginia Johnson conducted some of the first
extensive research studies about sexuality in the latter half of the twentieth century. One finding is important for understanding the nature
of our sexuality as men. That is that male infants, in the womb, have
regular erections—so do male infants after birth. Our sexuality is as
much a part of us as breathing, our need for food, our need for love.
Through it, we learn one of the deepest patterns embedded within
nearly all life forms on Earth. Through it, we can also experience the
joy of joining with another human being in one of the most intimate
and pleasurable acts ever known. But, this deeply ingrained sexuality
within men expands itself outward and becomes much more than simply a form of human procreation, enjoyable sharing, or deep intimacy.

Our sexual vitality flows through everything we do, infuses our work, helps us create new forms of work, play, and intimacy. It is an essential element in our response to the touch of the world upon us, and it is intimately connected to our capacity for imagination. Testosterone, research has shown, is an important neural chemical, not just a sexual hormone. It has many impacts in the central nervous system and on the functioning of the brain. Men enjoy watching women, in part, because it immediately stimulates their production of testosterone, which stimulates their imagination, which stimulates more testosterone, which stimulates . . . well, it just keeps going on.

This increase in male vitality then infuses everything a man does throughout the day. Physical agility increases, energy levels are enhanced, and the brain, infused with tremendous amounts of testosterone, becomes more mentally alert and imaginative. A study at the Max Planck Institute in Germany in 1974 revealed that three-fourths of the men who were shown a mildly erotic film experienced significant increases in their blood levels of testosterone. These high testosterone levels were found in another study to, not surprisingly, increase resistance and immunity to many diseases. There is a reason why men are biologically driven to look at those they consider sexually attractive—it stimulates testosterone production in the body and brain.

When androgen levels fall or the androgen/estrogen ratio is skewed too far, a great many things are affected. Many of the sexual problems that men struggle with can be directly traced to the high levels of estrogenic chemicals in the environment. Besides low free testosterone levels and imbalances in the androgen/estrogen ratio, the most common problems are infertility, erectile dysfunction or impotence, prostatitis, and benign prostatic hyperplasia (BPH).

Many of the plants already discussed in this book are good for these conditions, a few others are specific. The more healthy the testes, adrenals, prostate gland, and circulatory system are, the better the sexual health of a man, and the more energetic the production of androgens.

Infertility

Generally, *infertility* in men refers to either low sperm counts (oligo-spermia) or comatose sperm—sperm whose motility or movement is impaired. There are a number of plants, supplements, and foods that have been found to be helpful for these conditions, many of them in clinical studies or trials.

There are four plants and one combination of medicinal plants that seem to be the strongest for promoting sperm production and sperm motility. These are Chinese dogwood, tribulus, speman, and ginseng.

Natural Care for Infertility

Suggested dosage for two to six months:

Chinese dogwood: Tea daily

Tribulus: 250 milligrams three times per day

Speman: Two tablets three times per day

Panax and tienchi ginseng tincture: Up to one-third teaspoon per day

L-carnitine: Five hundred to one thousand milligrams per day

L-arginine: Five hundred to three thousand milligrams per day

Vitamin C: Five hundred to one thousand milligrams per day

Zinc: Twenty to forty milligrams per day

Vitamin B: Supplement daily

Chinese Dogwood (*Cornus officinalis*)

Family: Cornaceae

Part Used: Fruit

Collection and Habitat: Chinese dogwood, also called Japanese cornel, is an ornamental tree, much like our American dogwoods. It grows naturally throughout eastern China and Japan and has been planted as an ornamental throughout much of the rest of the world. The fruit is harvested when ripe. It should have an orange color and sour taste, a bit like a cross between a cranberry and a chewy orange candy.

Actions: Chinese dogwood fruit, called *Fructus corni* or Shan zhu yu in Chinese medicine, has been used for several thousand years as a tonic/stimulant for the kidneys/urinary system and as a tonic for the male reproductive system. The bark is a febrifuge (lowers fevers) and is often used for malaria. The bark of many other species of dogwood is used for malarial conditions as well; however, with this species, the fruits are actually favored.

The fruit is usually dried and used as a tea for: impotence, lack of sexual desire, incontinence, frequent urination, tinnitus, vertigo, hair loss, arthritis, and diabetes. Interestingly, this collection of physical problems are all associated with lowered or altered testosterone levels and poor blood circulation, which itself is linked to altered androgen levels.

About Chinese Dogwood: Many botanists consider Chinese dogwood to be much the same as our American dogwood *(Cornus florida)*, and some practitioners consider the two medicinally interchangeable. However, the only specific studies on sperm motility have occurred with the Asian species.

The current interest in the plant has been stimulated by its long standing use for several thousand years as a male fertility agent, usually as a tea, in both Japan and China. While limited, those Western-style studies that have been conducted on dogwood are highly promising. Regular consumption of an infusion (a strong tea) of dogwood fruit has consistently resulted in better sperm motility, generally increasing movement by as much as 68 percent. One particular chemical constituent of the fruit (as yet identified only as C4) has been isolated and found to be the most potent, enhancing motility 120 percent. Other studies have found that cornus increases blood flow to the kidneys and spleen and that the fruit enhances the antioxidant defenses of the heart's vascular endothelial tissue.

Suggested Dosage: Prepare an infusion by letting an ounce of the dried fruit steep in a pint of hot water for 20 minutes. Begin with one cup per day and slowly increase to three per day by the end of one week. Add honey if desired; the herb is somewhat sour.

Cornus can be somewhat hard to find. The Internet and Chinese herb suppliers are the best sources. See the Resource Section of the book for suppliers.

Contraindications and Side Effects: Do not use if there is blood in the urine or painful urination.

Herb/Drug Interactions: None known.

Tribulus *(Tribulus terrestris)*
About Tribulus: Tribulus was extensively discussed in chapter 4. Please refer to that chapter for more data on the plant. I include here only the material directly bearing on infertility.

Specifics for Infertility: Each testicle contains some five hundred convoluted somniferous tubules which, if laid end to end, would stretch 750 feet. Inside these tubules are the Sertoli cells that make both androgen binding protein and sperm. Androgen binding protein calls both testosterone and DHT to wherever it is located in order to concentrate androgens in a specific place. It is concentrated in the Sertoli cells and the epididymis, the long structure at the back of each testicle. It takes sixty-four days for the Sertoli cells to make sperm, which they do in sixteen-day intervals. Immature sperm cells, which are called spermatogonia, mature in sequence into spermatocytes, spermatids, and then into spermatozoa (aka sperm).

Tribulus is specific to both the Sertoli and Leydig cells of the testes. It causes the hypothalamus to release more luteinizing hormone (which stimulates the Leydig cells to produce more testosterone), increases the density of the Leydig cells (thus creating more cells to make testosterone), increases the levels of androgen binding protein, which increases the amount of testosterone and DHT in the Sertoli cells and epididymis (which increases the efficiency of the maturation of sperm), increases the numbers of spermatogonia, and increases the spermatogonia's transformation into spermatocytes and spermatids. This results in enhanced fertility in the men who take the herb.

As discussed previously in chapter 4, clinical study has found that from 50 to 80 percent of men using standardized preparations of tribulus experience significantly improved sperm production and motility. One study noted that taking five hundred milligrams three times a day for sixty days significantly increased sperm production for men diagnosed with idiopathic oligozoospermia (men who show *no* sperm in the semen from no discernable cause). Libido, erection, ejaculation, and orgasm all increased significantly for 80 percent of the men. Another, double-blind, placebo-controlled trial showed significant increases in sperm motility with corresponding decreases in immotile sperm. Numerous other studies have shown similar outcomes. Tribulus has been found to increase levels of leutenizing hormone, follicle stimulating hormone (FSH), DHEA, and interestingly, estradiol in women and testosterone in men but not vice versa. This indicates it is a general reproductive system adaptogen and tonic, rather than specific to gender.

Suggested Dosage: Tribulus is available under a number of brand names, including Tribestan, Trilovin, Libilov, and so on, and can be easily found on the Internet and in many health food stores. The usual dosage for infertility is between 250 and 500 milligrams a day for two to three months (or as directed).

The fruits themselves may also be used (as they traditionally have been for millennia) as an infusion or decoction of the powdered fruits: 1.5 to 3 grams daily.

Side Effects and Contraindications: The plant itself is not known to cause adverse reactions in people, and there are no known contraindications for use. Sheep and goats, however, do not respond well to the herb. Occasionally the plant can be infected with a fungus while in storage. This can be avoided if you harvest the plant yourself or if you buy a commercial, standardized preparation.

Herb/Drug Interactions: None known.

Speman

Speman is an herbal combination long used in traditional Indian (Ayurvedic) practice. It contains: *Orchis mascula* (65 mg), *Lactuca scariola* (16 mg), *Hygrophila spinosa* (32 mg), *Mucuna pruriens* (16 mg), *Parmelia parlata* (16 mg), *Argyeia speciosa* (32 mg), *Tribulus terrestris* (32 mg), *Leptandenia reticulata* (16 mg), and suvarnavang (mosaic gold, 16 mg). A number of clinical trials have explored its use in a wide variety of conditions, including oligospermia (low sperm count), oligozoospermia (no sperm in ejaculate), asthenospermia (lack of ejaculate), necrozoospermia (dead sperm), prostatitis, and BPH. About half of the men who take speman show significant increases in sperm count and motility; many of their wives subsequently conceive.

Clinical studies have included as few as twenty-one men to as many as six hundred. In only one example, 307 men between the ages of twenty-two and forty-five were given two speman tablets three times per day for three months. After three months, half of the couples conceived. Speman has been found to be effective, as well, in treating people with prostatitis and benign prostatic hyperplasia in a number of clinical trials.

Speman has also been used in vivo and been found to stimulate mouse sexual activity and to protect mouse testes, epididymis, and adrenals from cadmium poisoning. This is interesting in that speman shows a general protective and tonic effect on the male reproductive system. It corrects imbalances but also prevents future damage.

Suggested Dosage and Availability: Two tablets three times a day for three months, repeat if necessary. Widely available on the Internet from Ayurvedic suppliers.

Side Effects and Contraindications: Less than 1 percent of people who take speman complain of short-term dizziness, which is the only known side effect.

Herb/Drug Interactions: The literature does not mention any at this point in time.

Asian Ginseng *(Panax ginseng)*

About Asian Ginseng: This species has been found in numerous studies to increase sperm production. This is discussed in detail in chapter 4, beginning on page 34. Please refer to that chapter for more detailed information.

Suggested Dosage: Asian ginseng can be taken as tablets, one to nine grams per day, or as a tincture. The tincture is prepared 1:5 in 70-percent alcohol. Normal (American) dosage range is: five to twenty drops per day of kirin (dark red) ginseng tincture and twenty to forty drops per day of white. Asians often consume it in much higher dosages. **Note:** For androgen replacement purposes, Asian ginseng should be used and *not* American ginseng. I generally prefer to combine Asian ginseng with Tienchi ginseng (see next listing). I use a combination of tienchi (tinctured 1:5, 70% alcohol) and Asian ginseng, half and half, taking one-third teaspoon per day in water.

Availability: Asian ginseng in many forms is widely available at health food stores and on the Internet.

Side Effects and Contraindications: Ginseng can be quite stimulating and should be used in small doses at first and the dosage increased once you are used to it. It can sometimes cause hypertension, especially with large, sustained doses, and is contraindicated for those with extremely elevated blood pressure. It can be used with care in mild hypertension and with oversight in moderate hypertension. Sustained overuse can cause insomnia, muscle tension, headaches, and sometimes heart palpitations. It may cause difficulty in sleeping if taken before bedtime. Because it affects androgen and testosterone levels, it should not be used by adolescent men.

Herb/Drug Interactions: Avoid ginseng use with warfarin (Coumadin), phenelzine (Nardil), digoxin (Lanoxin), or haloperidol (Haldol). Avoid hypoglycemic drugs, anticoagulants, and adrenal stimulants. Caution should be exercised in its use with MAO inhibitors. Ginseng may block the painkilling actions of morphine.

Tienchi Ginseng *(Panax notoginseng)*

About Tienchi: In a number of studies, tienchi ginseng has been found to increase sperm production. It is discussed in detail in chapter 4, page 39. Please refer to that chapter for more detailed information.

Suggested Dosage: 1:5 tinctures—30 drops (aka 1.5 mL or ⅜ tsp.) three times daily. In severe depletion conditions, may be increased to twice that dose but side effects should be monitored. **Note:** For male health, as an antifatigue agent, and for testosterone enhancement, I prefer to combine tienchi ginseng with Asian ginseng. I generally use a combination of tienchi (tinctured 1:5, 70% alcohol) and Asian, half and half, taking one-third teaspoon per day.

Side Effects and Contraindications: Although not commonly known, tienchi, in a small percentage of users, can produce allergic reactions. Generally, these manifest as some sort of rash: urticaria, red papules, skin itching, flushed skin. Very rarely there can be mild anaphylaxis, abdominal pain or swelling, or diarrhea. These are uncommon—about nineteen instances reported out of millions of users.

High doses of the herb can cause nervousness, sleeplessness, anxiety, breast pain, headache, high blood pressure, insomnia, and restlessness. The plant is a corticosteroidogenic herb, that is, it stimulates the production of catabolic steroids such as adrenaline and cortisol by the adrenal glands.

The use of tienchi ginseng should be discontinued at least seven days prior to surgery because it can lower blood glucose levels and can act as a blood thinner. It should not be used during pregnancy because its constituents can cross from breast milk into nursing children. (These conditions correct upon discontinuance of the herb.) It should not be used by adolescent men due to potential androgenic conflicts.

Herb/Drug Interactions: Do not use with blood-thinning agents or warfarin (may decrease the effectiveness of those drugs). It may and probably will increase the effects of amphetamine-like stimulants, including caffeine. Do not use with haloperidol, an antipsychotic, it may exaggerate the drug's effects. Tienchi may block the effects of morphine and its use with MAO inhibitors, such as phenelzine, may cause symptoms such as headaches, manic episodes, and tremulousness.

Infertility Supplements

There are five infertility supplements that have been found to help sperm production in men. They are arginine, carnitine, vitamin B complex, vitamin C, and zinc. **Note:** L-arginine and L-carnitine, as opposed to arginine and carnitine, are natural forms of those substances rather than synthetic pharmaceuticals. When buying supplements make sure that you buy the L- form of both carnitine and arginine as they are more effective.

L-arginine

L-arginine, an amino acid normally present in the body, has been found, in some cases, to significantly improve sperm motility and sperm count. Arginine is an essential amino acid that is needed for the replication of cells, making it an important nutrient in sperm production. It is a natural source of nitric oxide, which is crucial for erections (see the Erectile Dysfunction section, page 108). One study showed a doubling of sperm count in two weeks with the use of L-arginine. In another, 74 percent of 178 men with low sperm counts showed significant increases in sperm motility and production. The latter study used four grams of L-arginine per day.

Suggested Dosage: Take one or two five hundred milligram capsules up to three times daily. Arginine is present in large quantities in pine pollen, sunflower seeds, brazil nuts, almonds, peanuts, lentils, kidney beans, and soybeans. Liberal quantities in the diet can help increase arginine levels in the body.

Side Effects: L-arginine should be avoided in cases of shingles or herpes because it can exacerbate the outbreak of these conditions. It will not usually initiate an outbreak, but existing viruses can use arginine to enhance their replication. L-arginine can also affect blood sugar levels and diabetics should only take it under the supervision of a health care provider.

L-carnitine

The epididymis, the oblong structure connected to the back of the testicles, is the first part of the excretory ducts of the testicles and, like sperm, it contains extremely concentrated amounts of L-carnitine. Low L-carnitine levels directly cause low sperm motility and production. Increasing the levels of L-carnitine immediately increases sperm motility—the higher the levels, the higher the motility. In one study, taking one thousand milligrams of L-carnitine three times daily for three months was found to increase sperm count and mobility in thirty-seven of the forty-seven men who used it.

Suggested Dosage: Five hundred to one thousand milligrams three times per day.

Vitamin B Complex

A number of B vitamins have been shown to play a role in both sexuality and sperm counts. B_{12} deficiency, for example, leads to reduced sperm counts and reduced motility. Studies have shown significant increases in sperm count and motility when men were given from one thousand to six thousand micrograms of B_{12} daily.

Niacin, another B vitamin, can produce a flush to the skin very similar to the flush many people experience during sex. There is a dilation of capillaries and blood vessels and an increase of blood flow throughout the body. In vivo studies with stallions have shown that the B vitamin niacin increases their capacity to reach orgasm. Many people taking it also report increased enjoyment of sex. Vitamin B_5 has been shown to increase stamina and endurance and has strong effects on maintaining healthy adrenal glands, the source of most of the body's DHEA. Choline, another member of the B-vitamin family, has been shown to exert strong effects on sex. Choline is involved in the production of acetylcholine, which is the primary neurotransmitter that sends signals from the brain to muscle systems throughout the body. Some studies have indicated that choline supplementation increases sexual responsiveness, interest levels, and stamina. Taking a good B-complex formula regularly is important; you may wish to add one thousand to six thousand micrograms of B_{12} as well.

Vitamin C

Vitamin C has been found to directly promote sperm health and motility. Dietary vitamin C plays a significant role in protecting sperm from DNA damage. In one study, dietary vitamin C was reduced to five milligrams per day from 250 milligrams. The number of sperm with DNA damage increased to 99 percent, while the ascorbic acid levels in seminal fluid decreased by 50 percent. Vitamin C has also been found to increase sperm motility in smokers (who tend to have lower sperm motility). Daily intake of from two hundred to one thousand milligrams of vitamin C can increase sperm motility and sperm production and reduce agglutination or the clumping together of sperm. (If more than 25 percent of sperm clump together, fertility is severely impaired.) In one study, by the end of twenty-one days, the amount of agglutinated sperm in men taking Vitamin C had dropped to 11 percent. By the end of sixty days, all of the women whose men were taking Vitamin C had conceived, but none in a placebo group had done so. Vitamin C also increases testosterone production and improves the P450 system in the liver, which eliminates excess estrogen.

I prefer taking Vitamin C as an effervescent, nonacidic powder in water; it's kind of like Alka-Seltzer. It is much easier to take this way, and it is assimilated into the body much faster.

Suggested Dosage: Take five hundred to one thousand milligrams per day.

Side Effects: Vitamin C can cause stomach upset, flatulence, and diarrhea when taken in quantity. It is often prescribed "t.b.t." or "t.b.d.," meaning "to bowel tolerance" or "to bowel dose." As soon as your body gets enough vitamin C, it excretes the remainder. To take Vitamin C t.b.t., take it until symptoms appear and then back off slightly. This is your bowel tolerance dose.

Zinc

Every time a man ejaculates, he uses five milligrams of zinc. Zinc is highly concentrated in both sperm and seminal fluid, and frequent ejaculation can lead to zinc depletion, especially if the diet is poor. Deficiencies of zinc in men result in reduced libido, low testosterone levels, and low sperm counts. Zinc levels are usually found to be low in infertile men with low sperm counts. Increasing the levels of zinc in the body can have an immediate, powerful effect on sperm motility, production, and even testosterone levels in the blood. A number of studies have shown that zinc supplementation immediately and significantly affects sperm motility and production. Even in cases of long standing infertility (more than five years), zinc can have a powerfully positive effect within two months. One study resulted in pregnancy for 40 percent of the men's wives within two months of regular zinc use.

Suggested Dosage: Men over forty should take twenty to forty milligrams per day.

Foods for Infertility

There are a number of foods that have been found to help increase male sperm counts: oriental cashew nuts, garlic, and oysters.

Oriental Cashew Nuts (*Semecarpus anacardium or Anacardium occidental*)

Family: Anacardiaceae

Parts Used: The nut, although the fruit (which is delicious) and the juice of the fruit have both been used medicinally as well.

Collection and Habitat: The oriental cashew tree grows throughout India and parts of China. It produces a fleshy receptacle, often referred to as an apple, at the end of which the kidney-shaped nut grows. There is an outer shell, ashen in color, and an inner shell covering the nut. Between these two shells is a highly caustic, flammable oil. (The tree is related to poison ivy.) Extreme caution must be exercised to avoid oil contact with the skin during harvest and processing of the nut.

Actions: Nutritive, cardiac tonic, mild aphrodisiac.

About Oriental Cashew Nut: In India, the Oriental cashew is commonly known as the "marking" nut because the sap of the tree (and sometimes the juice of the nut) has been traditionally used to make an indelible ink. In traditional Ayurvedic medicine, the nut kernel is considered to be a nutritive, digestive tonic, cardiac tonic, and respiratory stimulant. In Unani practice, it is used for polyuria (excessive secretion of urine), for improving memory, and as an aphrodisiac. It is common in folk medicine around the world to find the cashew used as a mild aphrodisiac and sexual stimulant for men. Interestingly, some clinical studies are beginning to bear this out.

Two human trials were conducted with Oriental cashew using the cotyledon—the first sprouting leaves of the germinating nut. An infusion using 2.4 grams of the dried cotyledon was prepared and taken by twenty and thirty-two men for fourteen and sixty-eight weeks, respectively. Improvements were seen in fertility, sperm motility, and sperm production.

Suggested Dosage: Eat the nut as often as desired as a regular part of the diet.

Side Effects and Contraindications: Nut sensitivities. Otherwise no side effects or contraindications are known.

Garlic (Allium sativum)

As discussed previously in chapter 6, Garlic has a long reputation as a sexually supportive food for men. Part of this is attributable to its reliable ability to reduce high blood pressure and improve blood flow. Garlic also stimulates the entire male hormonal system, thus increasing testosterone production and enhancing libido. There is some indication as well that it improves sperm production. One in vivo trial with mice showed a significant increase in sperm production merely from adding garlic juice to their food. For this and many other reasons, it makes sense to add garlic to the diet regularly and often.

Herb/Drug Interactions: Avoid if you are taking anticoagulants, paracetamol (acetaminophen), or chlorpropamide.

Oysters

Oysters have long been considered an aid to sex. The reason is that oysters concentrate zinc to high levels in their bodies. Zinc is, perhaps, the most essential trace mineral for the production of healthy sperm and one of the most important minerals to male health. One hundred grams, about four ounces, of oysters contain 150 milligrams of zinc. Eat as often as desired.

Things to Avoid

Cottonseed oil should be strongly avoided by men with infertility problems. The normal cautions about estrogenic plants also apply.

Cottonseed Oil

Men who regularly use raw cottonseed oil have been found to possess low sperm counts and eventually experience, if they do not stop, a total failure of the testes to produce sperm. This is because cottonseed oil contains a powerful male anti-fertility compound called gossypol, which strongly inhibits sperm production. Make sure that whatever you are eating does not contain cottonseed oil (it is often found in solid cooking oils).

Estrogenic Plants

As discussed in the last chapter, avoid licorice, black cohosh, and especially hops (as a supplement or in beer). All of these can interfere with spermatogenesis (the creation of sperm). Estrogenic substances such as hops interfere with the production of FSH or follicle stimulating hormone. In men, FSH supports the function of the testes Sertoli cells, which in turn, supports many aspects of sperm cell maturation and production. Any substance that reduces its production causes low sperm counts.

ERECTILE DYSFUNCTION

Some thirty million American men—about one-third of the sexually active male population—have been estimated to suffer some form of erectile dysfunction. When Viagra was released, one million prescriptions were filled the first year—a billion dollars in sales for the pharmaceutical giant Pfizer. Continued use, however, has also brought recognition of its side effects. Within five months, the U.S. Food and Drug Administration confirmed that sixty-nine people who had been using Viagra had died; forty-six of the deaths were related to cardiovascular disease, exacerbated, many felt, by the drug. Although there may be a place for Viagra, there are a great many natural approaches to treating impotence, the majority which have few or no side effects. One of the advantages of natural alternatives is that, in the long run, they can correct the underlying causes of many forms of erection problems. Viagra cannot, it must be taken forever (a common problem with pharmaceuticals).

There are a number of causes of erectile dysfunction, but four of the most prevalent are:

- estrogens or estrogen mimics in the environment or diet
- pharmaceuticals (can cause erection problems)
- atherosclerosis of the penile artery (basically fat-clogged arteries)
- diabetes-related high blood sugar levels, which cause a narrowing of the blood vessels

It is thought by a number of researchers and clinicians that about half of erectile dysfunction problems come from atherosclerosis. Erection depends on a strong supply of blood to the penis, and with poor circulation to the extremities due to clogged arteries, there is often an insufficient supply of blood to produce an erection.

If you have erectile dysfunction, have a check up for high cholesterol levels and diabetes. Simple tests in any physician's office can easily determine the presence of either of these conditions. Also, check the side effects of any pharmaceuticals you may be taking, scores of them cause impotence. Sometimes, the problem is just that simple.

Natural Care for Erectile Dysfunction

Take the following herbs and other substances for two to six months:

Ginkgo: 30 to 120 milligrams three times per day of standardized herb

Tribulus: 250 milligrams two times per day

Muira Puama: 250 milligrams three times per day

L-arginine: 1 to 2 500-milligram capsules up to three times per day

L-phenylalanine: 100 to 500 milligrams per day

L-tyrosine: 100 to 500 milligrams per day

L-choline: 1 to 3 grams per day

Zinc: 20 to 40 milligrams per day

Ginkgo (Ginkgo biloba)

Family: Ginkgoaceae

Part Used: Leaves

Collection and Habitat: The ginkgo is a tree indigenous to Asia (although it did grow in North America some millions of years ago before going extinct on that continent) and has now been planted as an ornamental throughout the world. The leaves are harvested in the fall when they turn from their normal green to a rich, ripe gold.

Actions: Ginkgo is a vasodilator, relaxant, anti-inflammatory, antimicrobial, and a cardiac and cerebral circulatory stimulant. Scores of studies have been conducted on ginkgo for use in stimulating peripheral circulation and improving blood flow in the brain, legs, and penis. Many of these have been double-blind, placebo, crossover trials. All of them have shown ginkgo's effectiveness.

Ginkgo has gained its modern reputation for helping the memory problems that sometimes occur with aging. Numerous clinical trials have shown that it stimulates blood flow in the brain, helping to alleviate forgetfulness and other memory disorders. However, ginkgo has a much larger range of action. It has been shown to be very effective in the treatment of heart disease and stroke, peripheral arterial insufficiency, eye disease, and impotence. Basically, ginkgo is effective any place in the body where there are problems from insufficient blood flow. This holds true as well for insufficient blood flow to the penis. Half to three-quarters of the men in various clinical trials have regained the ability to have regular erections after ginkgo use. In one trial, sixty men who had not reacted to injections of papaverine (a potent erectile stimulant) were given sixty milligrams of ginkgo daily for twelve to eighteen months. Blood flow improved after six to eight weeks of use, and after six months, 50 percent of the men had regained their ability to have erections. Another study explored the use of eighty milligrams of ginkgo three times a day by fifty men with dysfunction due to arterial insufficiency. The group was split into those who could achieve erection after injection of a drug (twenty men) and those that could not (thirty men). After six months of ginkgo use, the twenty men in the first group could achieve erections independently, as could nineteen of the men in the second group. Another trial found that after taking ginkgo for nine months, 78 percent of the men reported significant improvement in their ability to achieve erections. Ginkgo has even been found to help restore erections when the cause of dysfunction is from antidepressant pharmaceuticals. *For long term resolution of erection problems from arterial insufficiency, ginkgo is one of the primary herbs to use.* For short term, immediate gratification, potency wood and tribulus are more effective.

Suggested Dosage: The active constituents in ginkgo that help are considered to be present in insufficient quantities in the whole plant, so standardized extracts or capsules that concentrate them are generally suggested for use. Fifty pounds of ginkgo are used to make one pound of standardized extract. Usually the extracts contain at least 24 percent ginkoflavonglycosodes—what researchers consider to be the active constituent of the plant.

The suggested dosage is 60 to 240 milligrams per day. Improvement can usually be felt in two months, but restoration of regular erection ability can often take six months of regular use. Ginkgo's effectiveness has been found to increase when used with L-arginine and magnesium.

Side Effects and Contraindications: There is sometimes sensitivity to ginkgo preparations. Caution should be used if you are taking antithrombotic medications. Uncommonly, side effects can include mild gastrointestinal upset or headache and, very rarely, allergic skin reactions. In very large doses, ginkgo can cause diarrhea, irritability, and restlessness.

Herb/Drug Interactions: Ginkgo should not be used with anticoagulants such as aspirin and warfarin. Discontinue use seven days prior to surgery. Do not use with thiacide diuretics or trazodone.

Muira Puama *(Ptychopetalum olacoides; P. uncinatum and P. guyanna are considered interchangeable)*

Family: Olacaceae

Parts Used: All parts of the tree are used, most commonly the bark.

Collection and Habitat: Muira puama, native to the Brazilian Amazon, is a bush or small tree that grows to fifteen feet in height. Usually the bark is used medicinally; it can be harvested whenever needed.

Actions: Aphrodisiac, antirheumatic, antistressor, antidysenteric, central nervous system stimulant, nervine, neurasthenic (helps nervous debility and lack of strength). Reduces nerve pain, nerve paralysis, and hysterical stressed states.

About Muira Puama: Muira puama (aka potency wood) is native to Brazil and has a long history of use as an aphrodisiac and nerve stimulant in South American medicine. It was "discovered" by the Western world in the mid-nineteenth century and rose to prominence in the early twentieth. It has been a regular part of medical practice in England, France, and Germany since that time.

Muira puama seems to possess a consistently strong activity as an antirheumatic and neuromuscular tonic, helping alleviate muscle and joint pain. However, the primary benefits in erectile dysfunction are that it strongly relaxes and calms the body (which reduces stress effects on sexual arousal while promoting blood flow to the penis). This action in turn stimulates sexual arousal, erection, and central nervous system activity. These effects have been borne out in clinical use and trial.

In one clinical trial, 262 men with low libido and the inability to maintain or have an erection were given 1 to 1.5 grams of muira puama extract. After two weeks, 62 percent of the men experienced a return of libido, and 51 percent (132) had noted significant help with erectile function. Another trial found positive benefits for men with sexual asthenia (fatigue, loss of strength, or lack of sexual vitality, all of which are typical signs of low testosterone levels or androgen/estrogen imbalance). One hundred men complaining of impotence or lack of libido, or both, took part in the trial, ninety-four completed it. Sixty-six percent of the couples reported significantly increased frequency of intercourse, stability of erection was restored for 55 percent of the men, 66 percent reported reduced fatigue, and 70 percent reported an intensification of libido. Sleep improvement and increased morning erections were reported by many of the men.

The reasons for muira puama's actions are unknown, however the plant does contain a number of plant steroids such as beta-sitosterol, which has a normalizing and enhancing activity on male hormone activity. The herb has shown the strongest effects when the cause of erectile dysfunction is not psychosomatic and is caused more by fatigue and stress.

Suggested Dosage: Muira puama has been used for hundreds of years in the Amazon River region as a tea to help men with sexual dysfunction. However, a number of clinicians feel that the most effective form of the herb is as a tincture, one to three milliliters (¼–¾ tsp.) two times daily. The suggested daily dosage of the powder is 1 to 2.5 grams per day (about ½ to 1¼ teaspoons) or 1000 to 2500 milligrams of the encapsulated herb.

Side Effects and Contraindications: None noted.

Herb/Drug Interactions: None currently known.

Tribulus (Puncture Vine)

Tribulus is discussed in detail at the end of chapter 4. It has been found effective in a number of studies for helping stimulate erection. In one study, of seven impotent men using one standardized tribulus 250-milligram tablet, three times a day for two weeks, four of the men experienced improved erection, including prolonged duration of erection after treatment had ceased. Another study with fifty-three men using three 250-milligram tablets twice a day for three months showed significant improvements in a majority of the men in sex drive, erection, ejaculation, and orgasm. Three studies on diabetic men with erectile dysfunction found increased erection and sexual intercourse in 60 percent. In another study, treatment with tribulus for as little as four weeks showed improvement in erection, duration of coitus, and postcoital satisfaction in fifty-six men.

Part of the reason for tribulus's effectiveness is that it is a potent hypotensive, which means that it lowers blood pressure by relaxing blood vessels. It also facilitates the actions of nitric oxide and acetylcholine in the penis, and it stimulates the production of DHEA in the body. More on tribulus can also be found in the previous section on infertility.

Suggested Dosage: Take between 250 and 500 milligrams of the standardized herb as tablets or capsules three times a day for two to three months (or as directed).

Yohimbe *(Pausinystalia yohimbe)*
Note: I am not fond of this herb because I think there are too many potential side effects if used without sufficient knowledge. I am including it because so many people do use it and I think that the side effects from the plant and its wide range of herb/drug interactions should be understood.

Family: Rubiaceae

Part Used: Bark of the tree

Collection and Habitat: Yohimbe is an African tree growing to 100 feet in height that is common in west Africa. The bark from the branches or sections of the trunk is gathered when needed and dried for use.

Actions: Alpha-2 adrenergic antagonist, central nervous system stimulant, vasodilator, and erectile stimulant.

About Yohimbe: Yohimbe is the bark of an African tree that has, for centuries, been used in traditional African medicine for fevers, leprosy, coughs, and heart disease and as a local anesthetic. Because it so powerfully can dilate peripheral blood vessels, it has come to be used for erectile dysfunction. Most of the clinical trials, however, have been conducted using an isolated constituent of yohimbe called yohimbine (hydrochloride) which is available only by prescription under the brand names Yocon and Yohimex. Many of the over-the-counter preparations of yohimbe herb have been found to contain very little, if any, yohimbine (which it normally should have at about 7000 parts per million). If you do decide to use this herb buy only from extremely reputable herbal companies and use with caution (see Side Effects and Contraindications).

Suggested Dosage: Tincture: five to ten drops three times per day. Powdered yohimbe bark: one or two capsules per day. The standardized dosage of the isolated fraction, yohimbine hydrochloride, is fifteen to twenty milligrams per day, although a number of trials have shown that forty to forty-five milligrams per day may be a more effective range.

Side Effects and Contraindications: NOTE: This herb is best used under the supervision of a qualified health care practitioner.

Most of the side effects listed here are from the use of the purified extract, yohimbine. Some of these side effects are from extremely high doses (more than 200 mg) given either orally or intravenously. Side effects seem to be an inevitable occurrence when plant constituents are removed from their natural setting. Most plants contain numerous other components *whose only known actions* are to counter the side effects of their more powerful neighbors. Very few studies have been done on yohimbe toxicity as opposed to the toxicity of purified yohimbine. However, you should be aware of these possible problems before you consider using this herb or its isolated fraction.

Side effects include anxiety, elevated blood pressure, exanthema (skin eruptions), excitatory states, nausea, sleeplessness, tachycardia (rapid heart rate), tremors, and vomiting. Moderate to extreme overdosage can cause salivation, extreme pupil dilation, lowered blood pressure, cardiac disorders, hallucination, and death.

Yohimbe and yohimbine extract should not be used by people who have anxiety, manic-depressive states, depression, schizophrenia, panic disorder, nervous disorders, low or high blood pressure, heart disease, pregnancy, and peptic ulcer or by people who are taking numerous medications (see Herb/Food/Drug Interactions below). The German Commission E Monographs note, without explanation, that the herb is contraindicated in liver and kidney disease. This commonly has been repeated in various texts such as the Physicians' Desk Reference for Herbal Medicines. I have been unable to find a rationale for this in the literature.

Herb/Drug/Food Interactions: There are many. Amphetamines, cocaine, ephedrine, epinephrine, chlorpromazine, promazine, chloprotixene, phenoxybenzamine, and phentolamine all can increase the toxicity of yohimbine and presumably yohimbe. Clonidine and reserpine can decrease anxiety caused by yohimbine and presumably yohimbe. Metoprolol, penbutolol, and propranolol protect against toxicity of yohimbine in animal studies. Tricyclic antidepressants, including imipramine, clomipramine, and amitriptyline, can produce hypertension when taken with yohimbine and possibly yohimbe.

Yohimbe can reduce the drug absorption and bioavailability of brimonidine, but it enhances the actions of bupropion and fluvoxamine. Do not take yohimbe or yohimbine with liver, cheese, red wine, or decongestants.

Toxicity: A dose of twelve milligrams of yohimbe can induce a hypertensive crisis if taken with tricyclic antidepressants. A dose of ten milligrams can induce mania in manic-depressive states. A dose of fifteen milligrams has been associated with bronchospasm.

Supplements for Erectile Dysfunction

There are five supplements that have been found to help erectile dysfunction: L-arginine, L-phenylalanine, L-tyrosine, L-choline, and zinc.

L-arginine

L-arginine is the physiological precursor for the formation of nitric oxide, which the body needs for erections to occur. The body converts arginine to nitric oxide during sexual arousal, and uses it to generate an erection. The nitric oxide dilates and relaxes the blood vessels in the penis, allowing them to engorge with blood and the penis to become erect. The more sexually stimulated a man becomes, the faster the body's arginine is converted to nitric oxide. If the body is low in arginine, erections can be feeble or nonexistent. Increasing the supplementation of arginine alone has been shown to result in better and longer-lasting erections. Arginine is often used among animal breeders to enhance erections in bulls, roosters, and horses. More and more, research has shown that men can use the supplement with equally good results.

Suggested Dosage: Take one or two 500-milligram L-arginine capsules up to three times daily. Some researchers have suggested using six to eighteen grams forty-five minutes before sex. Others feel that lower doses of between 1.5 and 3 grams are sufficient. Taking the supplement just before sex (within 45 minutes) allows the body sufficient amounts of L-arginine to generate an erection in response to stimulation. Daily supplementation will bring arginine levels up over time. Foods that contain arginine should be added to the diet. (See the section on Infertility.)

Side Effects and Contraindications: L-arginine should be avoided in cases of shingles or herpes because it can exacerbate the outbreak. L-arginine will not usually initiate an outbreak, but existing viruses can use it to enhance their replication. L-arginine can also affect blood sugar levels, so diabetics should only take it under the supervision of a health care provider.

L-phenylalanine and L-tyrosine

These two amino acids are precursors to L-dopa, which stimulates both erections and sexual desire in people who take it regularly. Most are people with Parkinson's disease whose bodies have quit making L-dopa in sufficient quantities. The primary side effect of the supplements for men with Parkinson's disease seems to be heightened sexuality and a penchant for grabbing nurses.

Suggested Dosage: One hundred to five hundred milligrams of each supplement daily.

Side Effects: High doses of these supplements can increase blood pressure, especially if taken along with MAO inhibitors. Use with caution or under the care of a health care provider in cases of hypertension.

L-choline

A number of studies have shown that acetylcholine plays an essential role in the transmission of nerve impulses from the brain to the penis during sexual arousal. The tissue in the penis that engorges with blood is high in acetylcholine, and the chemical plays an essential role, along with nitric oxide, during erections. L-choline is now considered to be an essential nutrient, needed by the body to generate sufficient acetylcholine for neurotransmission in the brain and, importantly, crucial for sexual arousal. Studies have found that the supplemental use of L-choline increases the body's ability to generate erections.

Suggested Dosage: One thousand to three thousand milligrams (1–3 grams) daily.

Side Effects: High doses of L-choline may cause stiff or tight muscles in the neck or shoulders, tension headache, or mild diarrhea. Some clinicians suggest taking L-choline with Vitamin B_5 (pantothenic acid), which stimulates the health and activity of the adrenal glands and the adrenal output of male hormones. A few studies have found that the combination of choline and vitamin B_5 leads to longer and more pleasurable erections. Some companies offer combinations of vitamin B_5, choline, and arginine.

Zinc

Because zinc is so intimately connected to sexual health in men, it is essential to consider adding it regularly to the diet. A significant number of men with erectile problems have been found to be deficient in zinc. It is essential in the maintenance of testosterone levels in the body and the health and vitality of sperm. For more information on zinc, see chapter 5 (page 62).

Suggested Dosage: Twenty to forty milligrams daily.

Foods for Erectile Dysfunction

There are four good ones: ginger, garlic, fava beans, and ox-eye beans.

Ginger

Ginger has a long tradition of use as an aphrodisiac; in traditional Chinese medicine it is considered a sexual tonic. Contemporary research has shown that it does have a strong effect on helping prevent or reverse atherosclerosis, and it stimulates peripheral circulation as well. Because atherosclerosis of the penile artery is the cause of half the erectile dysfunction of men over fifty, any food that can reduce or reverse it has a place in the diet. Suggested serving: daily in the diet, use fresh grated in food or drink; one to two cups of ginger tea per day.

Garlic

Because garlic is so powerful for reducing atherosclerosis and thus helping improve blood flow to the penis, it should be liberally included in the diet (see chapter 6, page 82).

Fava and Ox-Eye Beans

There are now a significant number of clinical trials that show that adding foods high in soluble fiber, especially beans, to the diet regulates levels of blood sugar. Beans in general are important, but when impotence or erectile dysfunction are also problems fava beans are strongly indicated.

Fava and ox-eye beans (sometimes called velvet beans) contain significant amounts of L-dopa, an important prosexual chemical and dopamine precursor. L-dopa has the well-known side effect of increasing sexual interest and activity in anyone who takes it. It is also specific for helping create erections. Too much can cause a spontaneous persistent erection (priapism) that can sometimes be painful. Although neither bean contains enough to cause priapism by itself, healthy quantities of these beans can help stimulate erections while helping regulate blood sugar. Both have a reputation as aphrodisiacs, especially the ox-eye bean, which is a traditional aphrodisiac in Panamanian folk medicine. The sprouts of both fava and ox-eye beans contain even higher levels of L-dopa than the beans and are a good addition to salads. You can find these beans at many health food stores, and they can be easily ordered over the Internet.

Suggested serving: Eight to sixteen ounces of these beans three or more times per week.

Things to Avoid

Estrogenic plants, as already discussed, should be avoided, especially hops and hopped beers. Examine *all* pharmaceutical medications to determine if they can cause impotence.

Benign Prostatic Hyperplasia (BPH) and Prostatitis

Despite the major progress that has occurred in the biological sciences during the last 50 years, it is rather remarkable that we are about to enter the twenty-first century, and still the specific function of the prostate gland is unknown. Indeed the prostate is the largest organ of unknown specific function in the human body.

Dr. John Isaacs,
John Hopkins School of Medicine

The prostate, a walnut-sized gland that sits just below the bladder, wraps around the urethra—the tube through which urine flows. If the prostate swells, it can cut off the flow of urine, sort of like kinking a garden hose.

The more it swells, the slower and more problematic the urine stream. So . . . it takes awhile to get the urine going, the urine stream is weak, the urine dribbles on for a bit afterward, it takes more push to empty the bladder, and the bladder may only partially empty, making more trips to the bathroom necessary—usually in the middle of the night (nocturia). And to top it off, the stream isn't strong enough to fully open the tiny flaps at the end of the penis, and the urine stream shoots out in two directions. No matter how you aim, while one stream will go in the toilet, the other hits the wall, or the floor, or the seat. Your wife and friends begin to insist you sit down to pee. And it all used to be so easy.

Inflammation and enlargement of the prostate have both been around a long time. For hundreds of years, they were lumped together in a condition called strangury—a lovely, beautifully descriptive term—the *strangling* of the urethra, which causes the urine to emerge drop by drop. (It also referred to painful urination, I suppose from the expression on men's faces when they tried to go.)

Benign Prostatic Hyperplasia

There is currently a tremendous difference of opinion as to the cause of BPH. Conventional medical thought is that the accumulation of dihydrotestosterone (DHT) in the prostate is the problem. As testosterone enters the prostate, more than 95 percent of it is converted to DHT by the enzyme 5-alpha reductase. This DHT binds strongly to androgenic receptors in the prostate. Because it is the DHT that stimulates growth of the prostate when testosterone levels rise just after birth and at puberty, physicians have come to believe that DHT is the cause of its growth in middle age. There are a number of problems with this perspective, the most obvious being that growth of the prostate in middle age is occurring as testosterone levels in the body begin to *fall*, not rise. Prostate growth earlier in life only occurred during increases in testosterone levels.

Standard medical intervention for BPH takes a two-pronged approach. The first is to relax the smooth muscle contractions in the prostate through the use of alpha-blocker drugs. This allows the urine to flow more freely and alleviates some of the symptoms of BPH. The second intervention is to prevent the conversion of testosterone to DHT through the use of 5-alpha reductase blockers, usually the pharmaceutical Proscar (generic name finasteride).

Finasteride is usually of benefit only to men whose prostates are severely enlarged, from the size of a tomato to that of a grapefruit, which generally corresponds to Stage III or IV BPH. The drug needs to be taken for at least six months before there is any indication of effectiveness and usually one year for maximum effect. It does reduce DHT concentration in the prostate by some 80 percent, but the prostate only reduces its size by 18 percent in less than half of the men after one year of use. Only one-third to two-thirds of men (depending on the studies) show improvement in their symptoms.

Finasteride, in about 10 percent of men, causes impotence, decreased libido, and/or breast enlargement. It also decreases the levels of prostate specific antigen (PSA) that circulate in the blood. *Increased* PSA levels indicate the presence of prostate cancer about 70 percent of the time. This allows physicians to treat it before it spreads to other parts of the body. Finasteride interferes with the creation of PSA by normal prostate cells but not PSA created by prostate cancer cells. This means that men on the drug can show low levels of PSA even when they do have cancer. BPH is also considered to be a possible early indicator of eventual prostate cancer. Yet in at least one trial, men who take finasteride have been found to have an increased risk of prostate cancer.

Research is beginning to indicate, however, that the conversion of testosterone to DHT is not the reason behind inflammation of the prostate. Prostate growth, which in younger life is directly dependant on testosterone, begins to increase again in middle age exactly at the point when *testosterone levels begin to fall.* This later decrease in the body's levels of free testosterone is amplified by the simultaneous increase in levels of sex hormone binding globulin (SHBG), which binds up even more free testosterone and makes testosterone levels in the body fall even lower. For this reason alone, the assumption that DHT levels are the cause of prostate enlargement seems suspect. Several studies have even shown that men with enlarged prostates do not have higher levels of DHT than men without prostate enlargement. In fact, DHT levels in men with BPH were found to be slightly lower than in healthy men. Extensive studies have also been done to see if Chinese men, who generally have lower rates of BPH than American men, also have lower 5-alpha reductase activity in their prostates. The studies, which were designed to normalize the populations for numerous factors, found that Chinese and American men have the same levels of activity of 5-alpha reductase. The researchers commented that the studies indicate that the cause of BPH is environmental and dietary factors, *not* 5-alpha reductase activity. Something else is causing the epidemic of prostate enlargement in men.

Prostatitis

Prostatitis (inflammation of the prostate) is different than benign prostatic hyperplasia (BPH), although both are treated nearly the same with natural protocols. Prostatitis actually means an inflammation of the prostate gland, while BPH refers to a nonmalignant, abnormal growth in prostate tissue. Normally walnut-sized, during severe BPH, the prostate can literally grow to the size of a grapefruit. The degree of the growth in prostate tissue and the impact on quality of life are measured from Stage I (mild) to Stage IV (serious). Prostatitis is not usually accompanied by the same degree of prostate growth as that seen in BPH.

No one knows why most prostatitis occurs, less than 10 percent is caused by bacterial infections because it is difficult for bacteria to get into the prostate. Usually those that do are immediately killed by the body's immune system—causing a short-term, limited condition called acute prostatitis. Chronic bacterial prostatitis occurs when the bacteria are not killed, their population is only decreased, and they continually cause problems. Both of these conditions are usually caused by a urinary tract infection in which, for a variety of reasons, the urine backflows into the prostate, infecting it as well. This can be helped by using herbs and supplements for BPH while adding a urinary antibacterial such as uva ursi. If the bacterial infection is severe, the protocol for a urinary tract infection should be followed (see chapter 6). Other forms of prostatitis (chronic and asymptomatic prostatitis) occur from no known causes.

The prostate is just mildly inflamed, with or without symptoms. These more common forms of prostatitis respond very well to the same protocols that are used for BPH.

ESTROGEN AND THE PROSTATE

Very simply, the prostate contains two predominant types of tissues: stromal, which is composed mostly of smooth muscle and connective tissues, and glandular tissue, which is composed mostly of epithelial cells. Epithelial cells secrete prostate fluid and are also the site of most prostate cancers. Stromal tissues are the tissues that usually enlarge during BPH. (The glandular tissue enlargement that occurs during prostate cancer can cause the same symptoms as BPH. Both types of enlargement cause the urethra to squeeze shut.)

What researchers are discovering is that estrogens and androgens work together in the prostate to regulate its function. New findings show that while estrogens directly affect stromal tissues, they also condition the response of epithelial tissues to androgens. When androgen and estrogen levels alter, especially estradiol, the most potent estrogen, the evidence now strongly suggests that the prostate gland's tissues begin to grow in significantly different ways.

One study in Japan examined the levels of total testosterone, free testosterone, and estradiol in men who participated in a large, mass screening for prostate disease. Although free testosterone and total testosterone levels were found to be irrelevant to prostate disease, the levels of estradiol and the ratio of estradiol to both types of testosterone were found to be significant indicators of prostate disease. The higher the level of estradiol and the higher its ratio to both free testosterone and total testosterone, the larger the prostate was found to be. Another study at Harvard Medical School supported the Japanese research when it found the most significant indicator of BPH to be the level of estradiol in the blood. Researchers have in fact found that prostate tissue from men with BPH converts androgens to estrogens (primarily estradiol) at extremely high levels compared to healthy prostate tissue. This indicates that the enzyme aromatase, which converts testosterone to estradiol, has become highly activated in their prostates. This is a cause for concern in that it results not only in higher estradiol levels but also in much lower concentrations of testosterone in the prostate. Other studies have found that vitamin D is actually an important steroid hormone with powerful impacts on the prostate. When testosterone levels are low, vitamin D potentiates abnormal prostate tissue growth. With sufficient testosterone levels, it promotes normal prostate growth and cellular health.

Higher estradiol levels are a concern because stromal cells (the cells that usually enlarge during BPH) are the primary target of estrogens in the prostate gland. As androgen levels fall in the aging male body, the activity of estrogen receptor genes increases, leading, in many men, to increased stromal cell growth. Estrogen has been found to be a specific messenger molecule for the prostate's stromal tissue, initiating its growth. The impact of estrogen, especially estradiol, on stromal tissue has been found over and over again to be one of the primary factors in the development of BPH. During BPH, this estrogen-activated stromal tissue can increase up to two and a half times its normal ratio to other prostate tissues.

Increases in estrogen have also been linked with elevated levels of insulinlike growth factor, a protein that makes cells grow and prevents old cells from dying. High levels of insulinlike growth factor have been positively correlated with prostate cancer. Estradiol has been found to be the most potent estrogen that affects prostate tissues. It causes an eight-fold increase of in the amount of intracellularcyclic adenosine monophosphate (cAMP) in the prostate. This is a messenger molecule that is activated by hormones. Once activated, it initiates a wide range of activity within cells, including cellular growth. The level of cAMP is also directly correlated to the amount of PSA that the prostate cells release.

Androgens, especially testosterone, are converted into either DHT or estradiol through specific chemical pathways in the prostate. Part of the potential danger in focusing on 5-alpha reductase blockers is that they force testosterone and other androgens away from DHT conversion and into estradiol conversion, thus raising estradiol levels in the prostate. DHT, rather than stimulating prostate growth, tends to decrease estradiol levels and estradiol's impacts on prostate health. The primary factor emerging as most important in prostate disease is how much estradiol is either being taken in the diet (e.g., hopped beers) or how much estradiol is being made in the body or the prostate through the action of the aromatase enzyme. (Rises in estrogenic pollutants in the environment exactly parallel the increase in prostate disease in men.) Increased DHT levels, reduced aromatization, and reduced estradiol have all been correlated to better prostate health. *Because there is such controversy about the causes of prostate enlargement, you should explore the matter carefully and make your own decisions.*

NATURAL CARE FOR THE PROSTATE

Natural protocols for prostate disease are very effective. In Europe, they are the treatments of choice in 90 to 95 percent of cases. They work as well as they do, not because they interfere with the conversion of testosterone to DHT, but because they relax the muscle tissue in the prostate allowing urine to flow more easily. They also act as a prostate-specific anti-inflammatory, block the conversion of testosterone to estradiol, and normalize hormonal activity in the prostate. Natural treatment protocols are much cheaper than pharmaceuticals, do not have to be taken forever, tend to lower the risk of prostate cancer, and have few side effects when compared to pharmaceuticals. Because they possess such strong anti-inflammatory actions, these herbs are also specific for prostatitis.

Natural Care for Prostatitis and Benign Prostatic Hyperplasia

Suggested dosage for three to twelve months:

Nettle root: 300–600 milligrams twice a day

Saw palmetto: 160 milligrams of standardized extract twice a day

Rye grass pollen (Cernilton or an equivalent): 60–120 milligrams twice a day, especially for people with prostatitis

Omega-3 fatty acids: 1 tablespoon of flaxseed oil daily

Zinc: 50 milligrams per day

Nettle Root (*Urtica dioica*)

As discussed previously in chapter 4, nettle root has been used to treat both BPH and prostatitis in at least thirty clinical studies. Participants in the studies ranged from as few as twenty men to as many as 5,400. In men with Stage I–III BPH, nettle root consistently: reduced nighttime urination (nocturia), improved urine stream, decreased urine remaining in bladder after urination, decreased prostate size, and significantly lowered the score on the International Prostate Symptom Score (IPSS) questionnaire (this rates the degree of negative impacts the prostate inflammation is causing in urination in seven areas plus overall quality of life). A number of the trials were double-blind, placebo-controlled, crossover studies.

As only a few examples:

Sixty-one to eighty-three percent of 5,492 men who used 1200 mg of nettle root daily for three to four months found significant relief from BPH symptoms. In twenty-six men who used 1200 mg daily of a nettle root daily, prostate volume decreased in fifty-four percent and residual volume of urine in seventy-five percent.

Seventy-nine men who used 600 mg per day for sixty-eight weeks (sixteen months) found that urine flow significantly increased and urination time significantly decreased.

Twenty patients who used a combination nettle root/saw palmetto in a placebo-controlled, randomized, double-blind trial found their flow rate significantly improved over placebo. Their IPSS scores declined from 18.6 to 11.1 but with continued use continued to decline even lower to 9.8. The study found that continued use of herbs increases prostate shrinkage *over time,* improving prostate health the longer they are used. The same study compared 489 men with others using finasteride (Proscar) over a forty-eight week period and found that IPSS scores dropped similarly in both groups but with fewer side-effects in the men using herbal extracts.

Needle biopsies were taken in a number of studies to discover exactly what was happening to the prostate in men taking nettle root. Researchers found that nettle root reduced the activity of the smooth muscle cells in the prostate, caused a shrinkage of both the smooth muscle tissue and the epithelial or glandular tissue, and increased epithelial secretions.

Nettle root has been found to be consistently anti-inflammatory (both to the prostate and other tissues), to inhibit sex hormone binding globulin (SHBG), to inhibit DHT binding to SHBG, and to be antiaromatase (inhibiting the conversion of testosterone to estradiol).

The herb contains a number of powerful chemical constituents that are either unique to this plant, unique in these quantities, or in these combinations. Of note are histamine, formic acid, acetylcholine, 5-hydroxytryptamine, and various glucoquinones. Nettle is also exceptionally high in a number of vitamins and minerals, including zinc, and contains more protein than any other land plant.

Suggested Dosage: Capsule: Dosage ranges from 300 mg to 1200 mg per day of *nettle root* for three to twelve months in the majority of the clinical trials. Tincture: Dosage range is ¼ to 2 tsp daily of a forty-five percent alcohol/water tincture for one to twelve months.

Make sure in buying capsules and tinctures that you get the root and *not* the plant as each is used for different conditions. The root is often combined with saw palmetto. A significant number of effective trials have been carried out on this type of combination.

Side Effects: Mild side effects have occasionally been reported with the root, usually mild gastrointestinal upset. With the plant, only mild side effects are noted: skin afflictions such as rashes and mild swelling. The Physicians' Desk Reference for Herbal Medicines (PDR) lists a contraindication for the plant in cases of fluid retention from reduced cardiac or renal action. No contraindications are noted for the root.

Herb/Drug Interactions: May potentiate the actions of nonsteroidal anti-inflammatories.

Saw Palmetto (Serenoa ripens)

Family: Arecaceae

Part Used: Berries

About Saw Palmetto: Saw palmetto is listed in the German Commission E Monographs and the U.S. Physicians Desk Reference for Herbs as well as numerous herbals as being an antiandrogenic herb. This could easily raise concern for men wishing to restore androgenic levels in their bodies. However, those sources are incorrect. In actuality, saw palmetto is an *endocrine* agent, more specifically one that exerts steroidogenic normalizing actions on the prostate. Saw palmetto blocks both testosterone and DHT from binding to androgen receptors, but *it also blocks the action of estrogen in the prostate, interfering with the binding of estradiol to estrogenic receptors.* More technically, the herb suppresses expression of nuclear estrogen, progesterone, and androgen receptors in the prostate. Saw palmetto, in essence, successfully competes for both androgenic and estrogenic receptors in the prostate. This makes the herb a prostate tonic—which hormonal receptors it affects depends on how the prostate is malfunctioning. By interfering with the steroid hormones that are overactive, saw palmetto normalizes hormone action within the prostate gland and reduces cell proliferation and prostate growth. Although saw palmetto (and nettle root as well) does inhibit 5-alpha reductase, it and nettle root are both some 5,600 times less powerful than the drug finasteride (Proscar), lending considerable weight to the speculation that this action of saw palmetto is unrelated to its positive actions in the treatment of BPH. In fact, while saw palmetto has been found to lower the concentration of DHT in prostate tissue by as much as 50 percent, studies have shown that, at the same time, 5-alpha reductase activity in the prostate is unaffected.

Importantly, saw palmetto is also an anti-inflammatory through at least three different chemical mechanisms, which helps the prostate to decrease in size. It has been found to significantly reduce epidermal growth factor in the periurethral region of the prostate—the region of the prostate that surrounds the urethra as it comes down from the bladder. It is also an alpha-adrenergic receptor antagonist, which means that is relaxes smooth muscles throughout the body, including the prostate. These mechanisms alleviate the pressure of the prostate on the urethra, easing symptoms.

Saw palmetto has been used in at least twenty clinical studies ranging in size from fourteen to 1,300 men and has consistently shown effectiveness in reducing prostate problems. Of the men using saw palmetto in clinical trials, 80 to 90 percent report significant improvement in their prostate problems. Researchers have noted that for most men using the herb (89 percent) urinary flow increases, actual size of prostate decreases, and prostate symptom scores all decrease. *In general, the herb needs to be used for from forty-five to ninety days to produce benefits. The longer it is used, the more benefit is achieved.*

In one study, 505 men with Stage I to III BPH took 160 milligrams of saw palmetto twice daily for three months. Urine flow increased by 25 percent after ninety days, the amount of urine remaining in the bladder decreased by 20 percent, and the prostate reduced in size by 10 percent. Results on the International Prostate Symptom Score decreased by 35 percent. Another, four-month study with 1,334 men found that residual urine volume decreased by 37 percent and nighttime urination decreased by 54 percent. Half the men who had experienced painful urination before the trial reported relief.

Suggested Dosage: Standardized extract/capsules: Standardized to 85 to 95 percent fatty acids and sterols, take two 160-milligram capsules of extract twice a day. Powdered and encapsulated freshly dried berries: One to two grams one or two times per day.

Side Effects: Rarely saw palmetto will produce stomach upset and nausea.

Herb/Drug Interactions: None currently known.

Rye Grass Pollen *(Secale cereale)*

Family: Gramineae

Part Used: Pollen

About Rye Grass: Rye grass pollen has been used in Europe for prostatic, arthritic, and cholesterol problems for nearly fifty years with tremendous success. The pollen is generally sold in proprietary formulations under names like Cernilton or Cernitin. Interestingly, while 92 percent of the formulation is rye grass pollen, five percent comes from timothy grass *(Phleum pratense)* and three percent from corn pollen *(Zea mays)*. Corn pollen has been used as a longevity tonic for men and contains many of the same constituents as pine pollen.

The pollens are collected mechanically and processed through a two-stage process into pill form. Numerous clinical trials and hundreds of studies have shown this rye grass pollen combination to possess significant anti-inflammatory activity, to be a prostate tonic and normalizer, to lower cholesterol, and to be antiarthritic. Studies have consistently shown that this combination of grass pollens has a specific growth-inhibiting effect on prostatic epithelial cells and fibroblasts and that it is consistently effective in the treatment of BPH.

In one double-blind, placebo-controlled trial, fifty-seven men with BPH received either Cernilton or placebo daily. Seventy percent of the men in the Cernilton group reported significant improvement in symptoms, 60 percent of them reported improvements in bladder emptying, and most experienced a shrinkage of prostate tissues. Another double-blind, placebo-controlled trial with 103 men with Stage II or III BPH found that after taking 138 milligrams per day for twelve weeks, 69 percent of the men experienced relief of symptoms in six different categories. Another study with sixty men who took ninety-two milligrams for six months found similar outcomes.

Cernilton has been found to be as effective in the treatment of prostatitis as it has been for BPH. From 75 to 80 percent of men in clinical trials of Cernilton report relief from nonbacterial-related prostatitis. In one trial, men taking three tablets daily of a rye grass pollen extract experienced significantly reduced symptoms.

A limited number of studies have shown that this combination of pollens in Cernilton is effective in the treatment of rheumatoid arthritis as well.

Suggested Dosage: 60 to 120 milligrams two or three times daily. The dosage for rye grass pollen varies considerably. From 80 milligrams a day to 500 milligrams three times a day have been used by various clinicians and in various studies. The usual dosage range in clinical studies is three to six tablets or four capsules per day. Tablets are usually fifty to sixty milligrams.

Rye grass pollen is available under several commercial names Cernilton, Cernitin, and Prostaphil as several examples. Cernilton seems to be the most common (see the Resource section for sources).

Side Effects: This herb is contraindicated for those with pollen sensitivity.

Herb/Drug Interactions: None currently known.

Omega-3 Fatty Acids

In vitro studies have shown that omega-6 fatty acids actually stimulate prostate cell growth while omega-3 fatty acids inhibit it. This finding seems to transfer directly to people. Inuit/Yupik men who eat a lot of fish have significantly lower risks of prostate cancer than those who do not. One study with nineteen men found that an increase in omega-3 fatty acids for several weeks resulted in diminished residual urine in nineteen and elimination of residual urine in twelve; elimination of nighttime urination for thirteen; elimination of dribbling in eighteen men; increased urine stream in all men; reduction in the size of the prostate gland in all men; decreased fatigue and leg pain in all men; and increased libido in all men.

Suggested Dosage: Although you can buy omega-3 oil in capsules, perhaps the easiest way to take it is as flaxseed oil, one tablespoon daily. **Note:** Cold-water fish are high in omega-3 fatty acids. This includes mackerel, albacore tuna, sardines, salmon, and so on. If you do choose to eat salmon, try to get wild salmon. Most salmon sold in the United States are raised in pens and are nearly always treated with large quantities of antibiotics and growth enhancers.

Zinc

Zinc intake has been found to shrink the prostate and alleviate symptoms for men with BPH. Several studies have found that the use of zinc for as little as two months results in a decrease of symptoms of BPH. In one study with nineteen men, fourteen of them experienced shrinkage of the prostate as measured by palpation, x-ray, and endoscopy.

Interestingly, high levels of estrogen in the body interfere with zinc uptake in the intestinal tract. Not only do estrogens affect male sexual functioning but by lowering the uptake of zinc they also reduce male sexual functioning even further. Androgens, on the other hand, significantly enhance zinc uptake.

Suggested Dosage: Twenty to forty milligrams per day.

Things To Avoid

Hops and beer. The potent estrogen, estradiol, found in large quantities in hops, plays a powerful role in increasing prostate size and is strongly implicated in both BPH and prostate cancer. Hopped beer should be avoided at all cost. Some studies have found that beer consumption is directly related to prostate inflammation.

Other estrogenic plants such as licorice and black cohosh should be avoided as well.

Appendix
Ten-Week, Low-Fat Cleansing Diet

We eat the way we live. What we do with food, we do
in our lives. Eating is a stage upon which we act out
our beliefs about ourselves.

GENEEN ROTH

The following diet is exceptionally good as a general weight-loss plan if you want to reduce your body-mass index and waist circumference—two factors that are strongly linked to a higher ratio of estrogen to testosterone. Altering those factors will naturally increase the testosterone in the male body. One of the nice parts of this diet is that you can eat as much as you want, which helps reduce feelings of deprivation. The weight loss and the clearing of body sluggishness that occurs with this kind of diet are enhanced considerably if you immediately follow it with a juice fast for three to ten days. Energy and androgen levels will increase substantially. Two cleansing blends that I have had great success with are discussed immediately after the diet.

THE CLEANSING DIET

1. Drink four to six glasses of water every day. Do not use tap water.

2. Eliminate dairy products, eggs, and sweets.

3. Eat only *whole* grains (brown rice, millet, barley, oats, quinoa, and so on), organic beans, lightly steamed organic vegetables and fruit, and minimal amounts of wild or free-range meats. Tempeh and tofu are excellent. *Do not cook any grains with oil.*

4. Use only olive oil for cooking. Use no more than two tablespoons of oil per day. Do not use butter or margarine of any kind.

5. Drink all the fresh vegetable and fruit juices you like.

6. Do not use salt. Any other spices you wish to use are okay, as are small amounts of tamari and soy.

7. Do not use any caffeinated drinks (except green tea), alcohol, or recreational drugs during the diet. If you are a heavy caffeine drinker, instead of stopping cold turkey, go from coffee to black tea to green tea over a one- to two-week period of time.

8. Eat fruits first and by themselves. They digest rapidly and, when eaten with other foods, are held in the stomach where they can cause gas and intestinal upset.

9. Do not eat any fried foods.

10. Consider consuming a "green drink" each morning. Many of these are powdered and must be mixed into juice and blended. A fresh green drink recipe is described in chapter 6 (see Androgen/Adrenal Green Drink recipe, page 79).

FOOD LIST

Buy only organic, pesticide-free foods. This is important. The chemicals in non-organically farmed foods will be taken into the body, where they can have powerful impacts. You are working to lessen your toxin load, organic foods remove one common source of toxins that are often hard for the liver to process. This takes the load off the liver and allows it to work more efficiently in helping your body detoxify.

Fruits: Eat any fruits you wish.

Vegetables:

acorn squash	corn	red radish
artichoke	cucumber	rutabagas
asparagus	daikon	snow peas
avocados	daikon greens	spinach
beets	eggplant	string beans
broccoli	jicama kale	sweet potatoes
Brussels sprouts	red leaf lettuce	Swiss chard
burdock	romaine lettuce	summer squash
butternut squash	mustard greens	sprouts
cabbage	onion	tomatoes
carrots, raw or cooked	potatoes, red or white	turnips
cauliflower	parsley	turnip greens
celery	parsnips	watercress
collard greens	pumpkins	zucchini

Oil: Use olive oil for cooking. Flaxseed oil, because of its high levels of omega-3 oils, is a very good oil to use (uncooked) for such things as salad dressings.

Salad Dressing: Herbed vinegar, champagne, wine, or fruit vinegars only—combine with flaxseed oil if desired.

Seasonings: Any except salt.

Beverages:
Water: Filtered or artisan spring water. Do not use distilled water. Avoid all frozen concentrated juices.
Herbal teas: All are good, especially ginger, peppermint, and chamomile.

Meat: Fish from the sea, especially cold water fish. If you feel you want fowl, use only range-fed, pharmaceutical-free, organic chickens (or other birds). Wild meats such as venison or elk are excellent; if they are farmed they should be organic. Meat should be eaten only once or twice a week during the diet. **Note:** Salmon are almost always raised in pens in the sea. These fish are highly dosed with growth stimulants and antibiotics. They should be avoided. Eat only wild sea salmon. (Catfish are also farm raised.)

Bread: Use only sprouted-grain breads.

Cooking: Use only stainless steel, enameled, or earthenware cooking utensils. Never use aluminum.

Sweetener: Use pure maple syrup. It contains enough essential ingredients that it is possible to live on it for extended periods of time. Maple syrup supplies nearly all the essential vitamins and minerals necessary for health.

MEAL PLANNING

It is best to establish a routine for meals and a list of meals *before* you start on the diet. Cook a large pot of a grain of your choice and keep it in the refrigerator. This way if you get hungry, there is already something available.

Eat as much as you wish throughout the day. Fruit is good as a snack food. Have it available to eat whenever you feel hungry. It is helpful to get a good vegetarian cookbook and plan out a week's meals.

Sample Daily Menus

Breakfast: 1) Herbal tea, oatmeal with raisins and maple syrup. 2) Fruit salad. 3) Powdered or fresh Green Drink.

Lunch: 1) Vegetable soup, sprouted bread. 2) Rice and steamed vegetables with tamari.

Dinner: 1) Steamed vegetables or vegetable casserole, grain of choice, salad with herbed vinegar. 2) Steamed salmon with dill and lime, steamed asparagus, wild green salad with snow peas and radish.

Powdered Green Drinks

"Green drinks" have become more popular of late, and a number of types are readily available in health food stores and on the Internet. You can buy them premixed (follow directions on the container) or make them yourself. The one I make contains two parts each of spirulina, Siberian ginseng, nettle leaf, astragalus, turmeric, dandelion root, and milk thistle seed and one part each of chlorella, bladderwrack (a seaweed), burdock, and ashwaghanda. I add one-third cup of the powdered mixture to twelve ounces of apple juice, one tablespoon of flaxseed oil and blend, then drink. It is more effective if you begin blending the apple juice first, then add the oil and powdered herbs. Otherwise it clumps. This drink is just about as healthy a thing as you can take, and it is very filling, especially if taken at breakfast.

Things to Remember

1. It is normal to feel a sensation that is usually described as hunger no matter how much you eat in the early days to two weeks of this kind of diet. It is not actually hunger but the shift away from a high carbohydrate/glucose diet. During this time, your body will begin using more fat stores, shifting partially into ketosis (the burning of fat as a fuel, rather than glucose), to make up the calorie difference. By the end of the diet, most people generally feel increased energy, more mental alertness, and little hunger. They eat smaller portions, are highly relaxed, and have lower stress levels.

2. You may feel lightheaded. This is also normal.

3. Because eating is such a social event, it is normal to feel left out when others go out to eat. Go with them and convince them to go to a good health food restaurant. Order foods from the Food List (beginning on page 134) and that are light on oils.

4. When others order alcohol and you also wish to drink, order sparkling water with a lime in a champagne glass.

5. Emotional issues often arise during any change in eating patterns, especially when the body is using up its stores of fat. Remember

that this is normal, and make no major life decisions during this time. Remember, this, too, shall pass.

CLEANSING BLENDS ONE AND TWO

These two cleansing blends differ in their impacts. The first is strongly energetic and stimulating; the second is more tonic, nutritive, and gently supportive. The first is best used only short-term for fasts of up to ten days in length. The second is great for both short-term and longer fasts of ten to forty-five days. The first blend, which is also very good for colds and flu, is especially effective in stimulating the circulatory system. This helps support both the liver and kidneys in detoxifying the body. The second blend, often known as the Master Cleanser Diet (created by Stanley Burroughs), is a very good choice if you have not fasted before. It will give you enough energy to work and carry out daily tasks, most or all of the necessary bodily nutrients are provided, and it is very easy to make and use—there is no need for juicing at all. Some people simply fill a nipple-fitted, quart water bottle and carry it with them all day, drinking the blend whenever desired. **Note:** Do not substitute honey for maple syrup in Cleansing Blend Two; it is not as effective.

Cleansing Blend One

10 ounces spring water, hot
4–5 ounces fresh ginger root, juiced
1/4 fresh lime, squeezed into drink
1 tablespoon organic wildflower honey
1/16–1/8 teaspoon cayenne

Directions

Add juiced ginger, squeezed lime and its juice, honey, and cayenne to hot water. Prepare and drink three to six times daily, more if desired.

Cleansing Blend Two

The Master Cleanser Diet

10 ounces spring water, medium hot

2 tablespoons fresh lemon or lime juice

2 tablespoons pure organic maple syrup

$\frac{1}{16}$–$\frac{1}{8}$ teaspoon cayenne

Directions

Add squeezed lime or lemon and its juice, maple syrup, and cayenne to hot water. Prepare and drink three to six times daily, more if desired.

Ginger *(Zingiber officinale)*

Family: Zingiberaceae

Part Used: Root

About Ginger: Ginger possesses about 1 percent by weight of calcium, phosphorous, and iron. It is somewhat high in the B vitamins, particularly thiamine, riboflavin, and niacin. It also contains a fair amount of vitamin C.

Ginger is primarily a circulatory herb with pronounced effects on the heart and blood. It causes the blood vessels to relax and expand, thus lowering blood pressure and allowing the heart to beat stronger and more slowly as it pumps the blood throughout the body. This means that the blood is pumped more efficiently. Japanese researchers have found that blood pressure typically lowers 10 to 15 percent after ingesting ginger. Indian researchers have found that ginger is effective in lowering the cholesterol content of the blood. Dutch researchers have noted it to be efficient in preventing the blood from clotting, similar in effectiveness to aspirin. Ginger also soothes the stomach, helping to relieve indigestion and stimulate healthy digestion. It relieves gas, flatulence, and cramping and facilitates absorption of foods in the stomach.

A number of researchers have found that ginger is highly effective in alleviating motion sickness, nausea, and vomiting, being more effective than Dramamine, the usual drug of choice for those conditions. It has also been shown to be quite effective for morning sickness. Numerous studies have shown that ginger alleviates the symptoms of arthritis.

Ginger is a potent inhibitor of the inflammatory compounds known as prostaglandins and thromboxanes, which is one of the reasons why it so powerfully helps alleviate arthritic conditions. It is also a strong antioxidant and contains a protein-digesting enzyme (a protease) that appears to have strong impacts on inflammatory processes in the body.

Ginger is highly antibacterial with potent activity against a number of human pathogenic bacteria as well as the food-borne bacteria shigella, E. coli, and salmonella. Its antitussive (anticough) action rivals that of codeine, and it is a strong expectorant which helps move bronchial mucus up and out of the system.

Suggested Dosage: Start with a piece about the size of your thumb and work up. You can either grate the fresh ginger and then steep it in hot water for twenty to thirty minutes or juice it in a juicer and simply add the juice to the hot water. I usually juice it.

Many people start with about one ounce of juice in 6–8 ounces water and then increase the amount of juiced ginger as desired and as they become used to it. I prefer four to five ounces at this point, but I really like it spicy and I really enjoy the effects of ginger on my metabolism. I also save the juiced pulp and steep it in 6–8 ounces of hot water for a second cup later in the day. I find this to be as strong a tea as that from the original juice. Drink three to six times daily, more if desired.

Lime (*Citrus aurantifolia*) or Lemon (*Citrus lemon*)

Family: Rutaceae

Part Used: Fruit

About Limes and Lemons: One-quarter of a lime contains 4 milligrams calcium, 20 milligrams potassium, 2 milligrams phosphorous, 5 milligrams vitamin C, 0.25 milligrams sodium, 1 milligram magnesium, and varying trace amounts of iron, vitamin A, B-complex vitamins, germanium, tin, selenium, and zinc. Lemons are a bit higher in most of these constituents, mostly due to their larger size. Limes and lemons are strongly antibacterial and antimicrobial. They also contain (especially in the peels) compounds known as flavonoids, including rutin. These compounds affect vascular permeability. Essentially, they strengthen the walls of capillaries and blood vessels. This helps reduce the occurrence of varicose veins, for instance, and plays a role in preventing stroke and hemorrhoids. Limes are mildly anti-inflammatory and diuretic; they help increase urine production and flow. Limes (and lemons) also contain limonene that, while it helps dissolve gallstones, is also showing a great deal of promise in both preventing and treating cancer. It strongly enhances both phase I and phase II detoxification enzymes in the liver. This not only is effective in helping treat and prevent cancer, but is especially good for helping enhance the liver's ability to process the body's accumulated toxins. Limonene is specifically necessary for the parts of the phase II detoxification system that work through glutathione conjugation and glucuronidation. These two processes deactivate acetaminophen, nicotine, organophosphates (insecticides), various carcinogens, and a number of pharmaceuticals, thus protecting liver integrity.

Limonene is mostly present in the white, spongy inner pith (between the peel and the inner fruit) of limes and lemons. Because the peel and pith are so bioactive, it is more beneficial to squeeze the juice from a lime or lemon wedge into the drink, then drop the wedge in as well and let it steep.

Suggested Dosage: One-quarter fresh lime squeezed into glass and dropped into glass as well. Lemon can be used interchangeably, I just like the taste of lime better in Cleansing Blend One.

Cayenne (Capsicum minimum)

Family: Solanaceae

Part Used: Fruit

About Cayenne: Cayenne is extremely high in vitamin C, copper, and phosphorous; high in vitamin A; and a good source of bioflavonoids, potassium, and vitamin E.

Cayenne increases the body's metabolic rate, in some studies, by as much as 25 percent. This causes the body to burn more fat as fuel and makes cayenne especially helpful in increasing weight loss when taken during fasting. It also increases blood circulation, dilates capillaries, increases blood flow to outlying portions of the body, and lowers blood pressure. These actions make it especially useful during cleansing fasts. Cayenne is also a potent pain reliever. It contains capsaicin, a compound that stimulates the release of endorphins, the body's natural pain relievers. A number of studies have found it to be exceptionally effective in the treatment of cluster headaches and the pain of arthritis. Cayenne is also a powerful antiseptic and breaks up mucous throughout the respiratory tract and helps it move up and out of the system.

Because fasting can sometimes be accompanied by joint pain or headaches and is almost always accompanied by coldness in the extremities, cayenne's effects make it an excellent herb to use during a fast.

Suggested Dosage: $\frac{1}{16}$ to $\frac{1}{8}$ teaspoon per cup of water. **Warning:** Be careful that you don't get the cayenne on your hands. If you do, wash them thoroughly afterward. Otherwise, before you know it, you will rub your eyes or go to the bathroom and find yourself burning in whichever area you have touched.

Honey

About Honey: Honey is made from the nectar of the flowers of plants that is gathered by bees. Plant nectars contain sucrose, water, amino acids, proteins, lipids, antioxidants, alkaloids, glycosides, thiamine, riboflavin, nicotinic acid, pantothenic acid, pyridoxin, biotin, folic acid, medoinositol, fumaric acid, succinic acid, oxalic acid, citric acid, tartaric acid, a-ketoglutaric acid, gluconic acid, glucuronic acid, allantoin, allantoic acid, dextrin, formic acid, a wide range of vitamins and minerals, and other unidentified compounds.

The sugar in plant nectars is primarily sucrose, a disaccharide. Sucrose (most commonly experienced as white table sugar) is a double-molecule sugar that is made from one fructose molecule and one glucose molecule linked together. When bees harvest plant nectars, they hold them in their stomachs for transport to the hive. During transport, their stomach enzymes take the sucrose molecule and break it apart into glucose and fructose.

These two primary sugars in honey are monosaccharides (simple sugars) and, as a result, do not require additional processing by the body to be digested. White sugar, which is a disaccharide, takes considerably more work to be digested. Other than the sugar in fruits, honey, and the plant nectars it comes from, is the most ancient form of sugar concentrate that the human species has used.

Historically, honeys came from a profusion of wildflowers, whatever grew locally. It was exceedingly uncommon to have a honey gathered from a single species of plant, such as the alfalfa or clover honeys of today, unless that plant species existed in great abundance (as was the case with heather). Because of this, the wildflower honeys that humans have used throughout their evolutionary history have contained trace amounts of the medicinal compounds produced by a multitude of wild plants. Honeybees show a great attraction for many strongly medicinal plants, including vitex, jojoba, elder, toadflax, balsam root, echinacea, valerian, dandelion, and wild geranium. In fact, this includes almost any flowering medicinal herb as well as the more commonly known alfalfas and clovers. These plant compounds, although present in tiny quantities, remain highly bioactive.

Honey is not just another simple carbohydrate like white sugar is. It is composed of a highly complex collection of enzymes, plant pigments, organic acids, esters, antibiotic agents, and trace minerals. Honey, in fact, contains more than seventy-five different compounds. In addition to those already listed, it contains proteins, carbohydrates, hormones, and antimicrobial compounds. One pound of non-heather honey contains 1,333 calories (compared with white sugar at 1,748 calories), 1.4 grams of protein, 23 milligrams of calcium, 73 milligrams of phosphorus, 4.1 milligrams of iron, 1 milligram of niacin, and 16 milligrams of vitamin C.

The content of each of these substances varies considerably depending on which type of plants the honey is gathered from; some types of honey may contain as much as 300 milligrams of vitamin C per 100 grams of honey. Honey also contains vitamin A, beta-carotene, the complete complex of B vitamins, vitamin D, vitamin E, vitamin K, magnesium, sulphur, chlorine, potassium, iodine, sodium, copper, manganese, and a rich supply of live enzymes. It also contains relatively high concentrations of hydrogen peroxide, and many of the remaining substances in honey are so complex that they have yet to be identified. It has been found to possess antibiotic, antiviral, anti-inflammatory, anticarcinogenic, expectorant, antifungal, immune-stimulating, antiallergenic, laxative, antianemic, and tonic properties. Because honey increases calcium absorption in the body, it is also recommended for women in menopause to help prevent osteoporosis. In clinical trials, honey has been found to be especially effective in treating stomach ulceration (especially if caused by *Helicobacter pylori* bacteria), infected wounds, severe skin ulceration, and respiratory illnesses. A Bulgarian study of 17,862 patients found that honey was effective in improving chronic bronchitis, asthmatic bronchitis, bronchial asthma, chronic and allergic rhinitis, and sinusitis.

Honey is a reliable, stable source of vitamins and minerals. Although high in vitamins, fruits and vegetables tend to lose them over time. Spinach, for instance, loses 50 percent of its vitamin-C content within twenty-four hours of picking. Honey, on the other hand, stores its vitamins indefinitely. Wildflower honeys generally have the largest overall concentration of vitamins. Single-plant honeys tend to increase concentrations of one vitamin to the detriment of others.

Suggested Dosage: One tablespoon per cup of tea. Generally, raw, unprocessed, and unpasteurized wildflower honey should be used. Single-plant honeys such as those made from alfalfa and clover are generally from high-technology, monocropped fields that are doused with large amounts of pesticides and fertilizers. Use only organic wildflower honeys.

Side Effects and Contraindications: Occasionally, uncooked honeys can contain botulism spores that can be dangerous to children under one year of age. The human digestive system is more developed and able to deactivate the spores after about age one. In rare instances, people who are allergic to bee stings or who have pollen sensitivity may react negatively to honey. If you have a history of these kinds of allergic reactions, avoid honey.

Maple Syrup (Acer saccharum)

About Maple Syrup: Sap from the sugar maple is virtually the only tree sap still used in the United States. Originally, the members of indigenous cultures in North America, like many indigenous peoples, tapped a wide variety of trees—not only all the maples (6 species) and birches (6 species) but also butternut and hickory trees. These saps were used not only as syrups—made by boiling them down—but as tonic drinks, as medicines.

Maple is rarely used in contemporary herbalism, but early New Englanders often drank the fresh sap as a primary spring tonic. (From the time I spent living in Vermont, I find that many maple sap harvesters still do.) Maple sap, and the syrup that comes from it, is one of the most complete nutrient foods known. It is possible to live for many weeks without any adverse physical effects while eating only maple syrup. It is high in calories, calcium, potassium, phosphorus, and vitamin B_{12}. It also contains significant amounts of many other B vitamins and iron. Maple sap has traditionally been used, both internally and externally, as a general tonic, for skin conditions such as hives and stubborn wounds, as a kidney medicine and tonic, as a diuretic, as a cough remedy, for cramping, and as a blood purifier.

Because of its complex nutritional makeup, effectiveness as a general system tonic, and impacts on the kidney system, maple syrup is especially useful when used long-term for fasting.

Suggested Dosage: Two tablespoons in ten ounces of water daily as often as desired.

Resources and Sources of Supply

The Internet is a good source for everything. If you can't find something discussed in this book, try the Google search engine: http://www.google.com. If you begin using a large quantity of herbs, you might consider obtaining a resale license from your state (there is a minimal fee) and then setting up a wholesale account with an herb company. The prices tend to be somewhere between one-half and one-tenth of retail.

Pine Pollen

Although widely available in Asia, pine pollen has not yet caught on in the Western world. This is sure to change as it is used by more people. At the present, there are two major sources for the herb that I am aware of: one for tincture, one for tablets.

In my opinion, the best results for increasing testosterone levels with pine pollen come from the use of a tincture. Little of the tincture reaches the stomach, but rather is absorbed into the bloodstream fairly quickly through the mucous membranes of the mouth and throat. The supplemental use of the pollen powder in tablet form would be supportive overall.

Tincture

Woodland Essence
P.O. Box 206
Cold Brook, NY 13524
1–315–845–1515
www.woodlandessence.com

Tablets

The best source seems to be a seller on the Internet auction site eBay at this point in time. The seller is located in Canada but will ship to the United States and sells a product produced by the GuoZhen Company of China under the product line name New Era Botanicals. The quality appears to be good. Just go to http://www.ebay.com on the Internet and type in "pine pollen."

Pine pollen tablets and/or powder may also be available from the following suppliers.

Shen Clinic Chinese Herbs
1385 Shattuck Avenue
Berkeley, Ca, 94701
1–877–922–4732 (toll-free); 1–510–848–4372.

Bee Fit Herbs
4710 Yelm Highway
Lacey, WA 98503
1–888–842–2049
www.1stchineseherbs.com

Herbal Remedies
1–866–467–6444 (toll free in United States)
1–307–577–6444 (outside United States)
www.herbalremedies.com

General Herbs, Retail

Dandelion Botanical
5424 Ballard Ave. NW Suite 103
Seattle, WA 98107
1–206–545–8892
1-877-778-4869 (toll-free)
www.dandelionbotanical.com

Woodland Essence
P.O. Box 206
Cold Brook, NY 13524
1–315–845–1515
www.woodlandessence.com

Herbs, Wholesale and Retail

Blessed Herbs
109 Barre Plains Road
Oakham, MA 01068
1–800–489–4372 (toll-free)
1–508–882–3839
www.blessedherbs.com

Pacific Botanicals, LLC
4840 Fish Hatchery Road
Grants Pass, OR 97527
1–541–479–7777
1-541-479-7780 (fax)
www.pacificbotanicals.com

Starwest Botanicals
11253 Tradecenter Drive
Rancho Cordova, CA 95742
1–800–800–4372 (toll-free)
www.starwest-botanicals.com

Rye Grass Pollen (Cernilton)

Graminex
95 Midland Road
Saginaw, MI 48603
1–877–472–6469 (toll-free)
www.graminex.com

Japanese Dogwood *(Cornus fructi)*

1st Chinese Herbs
5018 View Ridge Drive
Olympia, WA 98501
1–888–842–2049 (toll-free)
1-360-923-0486
www.1stchineseherbs.com

Speman

Lynx Ayurvedics
P.O. Box 14-084
Hamilton, New Zealand
64–7–855–4555
www.world-lynx.com

Supplements

Seacoast Natural Foods
 1–800–555–6792 (toll-free)
www.seacoastvitamins.com

Life Extension Foundation
1100 West Commercial Blvd.
Fort Lauderdale, FL 33309
1–800–544–4440 (toll-free)
www.lef.org

Wholesale Nutrition
P.O. Box 3345
Saratoga, CA 95070
1–800–325–2664 (toll-free)

Hardbody Nutrition
1–800–378–6787 (toll-free)
www.hardbodynutrition.com

NOTES

CHAPTER 1: THE IMPORTANCE OF NATURAL HORMONE SUPPORT FOR MEN

1. James Hillman, *The Force of Character and the Lasting Life* (New York: Random House, 1999), 54.

CHAPTER 2: ANDROPAUSE

1. H. A. Feldman et al., "Impotence and its medical and psychosocial correlates: results of the Massachusetts male aging study," *J Urol* 15, no. 1 (1994): 54–61.

CHAPTER 3: ENVIRONMENTAL POLLUTANT IMPACTS ON TESTOSTERONE

1. Peter Montague, "The Challenge of Our Age," *Rachel's Health and Environment Weekly*, no. 447 (June 22, 1995): 2.
2. J. Toppari et al., "Male Reproductive Health and Environmental Xenoestrogens," *Environmental Health Perspectives* 104 (4): 741–803; Theo Colburn et al., *Our Stolen Future* (New York: Plume, 1995).
3. R. Bergstrom et al., "Increase in testicular cancer incidence in six European countries," *Journal of the National Cancer Institute* 88, no. 11 (1996): 727–33; J. McKiernan et al., "Increasing risk of developing testicular cancer by birth cohort in the United States," *Dialogues in Pediatric Urology* 23, no. 1 (2000): 7–8, cited in Colburn, *Our Stolen Future*.
4. Louis Guillette, "Impacts of endocrine disruptors on wildlife," Endocrine Disruptors and Pharmaceutically Active Compounds in Drinking Water

Workshop, Center for Health Effects of Environmental Contamination, April 19–21, 2000, http://www.cheec.uiowa.edu/conferences/edc_2000/guillette.html.

5. Ibid., 6.

6. Stephen Harrod Buhner, *The Lost Language of Plants* (White River Junction, Vt.: Chelsea Green, 2002), 96.

7. Guillette, "Endocrine Disruptors," 5.

8. Center for Environmental Studies, Tulane and Xavier Universities, "Environmental Estrogens Differ from Natural Hormones," p. 3, http://www.tmc.tulane.edu/ecme/eehome.basics/eevshorm/default.html.

9. Montague, "Challenge of Our Age," 3; W. Kelce et al., "Persistent DDT Metabolite p,p'-DDE is a Potent Androgen Receptor Antagonist," *Nature* 375 (1995): 581–85.

10. Montague, "Challenge of Our Age," 4; L. Gray et al., "Developmental effects of an environmental antiandrogen: The fungicide vinclosolin alters sex differentiation of the male rat," *Toxicology and Applied Pharmacology* 129 (1994): 46–52.

11. Gerald LeBlanc, "Are Environmental Sentinels Signaling?," *Environmental Health Perspectives* 103, no. 10 (1995): 888–90.

12. Colburn, *Our Stolen Future*, 85.

13. J. Ostby et al., "Perinatal exposure to the phthalates DEHP, BBP, but not DEP, DMP, or DOTP permanently alters androgen-dependent tissue development in Sprague-dawley rats," *Biology of Reproduction* 62 (2000): 184.

14. Ted Schettler, "Phthalate Esters and Endocrine Disruption," The Science and Environmental Health Network, p. 2, http://www.sehn.org/pubhealthessays.html.

15. Greenpeace, "Taking Back Our Stolen Future," April 1996, http://www.archive.greenpeace.org/toxics/reports/tbosf/tbosf.html.

16. Colburn, *Our Stolen Future*, 178.

17. Peter Montague, "Warning on Male Reproductive Health," *Rachel's Health and Environment Weekly*, April 20, 1995, p. 1.

18. Ibid., 2.

CHAPTER 4: PHYTOANDROGENS

1. Steven Foster and Yue Chongxi, *Herbal Emissaries* (Rochester, Vt.: Healing Arts Press, 1992).
2. Ibid.

CHAPTER 5: SUPPLEMENTS TO INCREASE TESTOSTERONE LEVELS

1. Jonathan V. Wright and Lane Lenard, *Maximize Your Vitality and Potency for Men Over 40* (Petaluma, Calif.: Smart Publications, 1999).

CHAPTER 6: ANDROGENIC FOODS

1. Garcilaso de la Vega, *Royal commentaries of the Incas and General History of Peru,* 2 vols., trans. Harold V. Livermore (Austin: University of Texas Press, 1966).

CHAPTER 7: TESTOSTERONE ANTAGONISTS

1. Eugene Shippen and William Fryer, *The Testosterone Syndrome* (New York: Evans, 1998).

BIBLIOGRAPHY

This is the general bibliography used for the material in this book. A listing of scientific and popular papers on specific herbs, foods, and supplements follows the general list.

Balch, James, and Phyllis Balch. *Prescription for Nutritional Healing*. New York: Avery, 1997.

Bensky, Dan, and Andrew Gamble. *Chinese Herbal Medicine Materia Medica*. Rev. ed. Seattle: Eastland Press, 1993.

Bergner, Paul. *The Healing Power of Garlic*. Rocklin, Calif.: Prima, 1996.

———. *The Healing Power of Ginseng*. Rocklin, Calif.: Prima, 1996.

Blumenthal, Mark, et al. *The Complete German Commission E Monographs*. Austin, Tex.: American Botanical Council, 1998.

Buhner, Stephen Harrod. *Herbal Antibiotics: Natural Alternatives for Drug-Resistant Bacteria*. Pownal, Vt.: Storey Books, 1998.

———. *The Lost Language of Plants*. White River Junction, Vt.: Chelsea Green, 2002.

———. *Sacred and Herbal Healing Beers: The Secrets of Ancient Fermentation*. Boulder, Colo.: Siris Press, 1998.

———. *Vital Man*. New York: Avery, 2003.

Chang, Hson-Mou, and Paul Pui-Hay But, eds. *Pharmacology and Applications of Chinese Materia Medica*. 2 vols. London: World Scientific, 1986.

Cherniske, Stephen. *The DHEA Breakthrough*. New York: Ballantine, 1998.

Colburn, Theo, Dianne Dumanoski, and John Peterson Myers. *Our Stolen Future*. New York: Plume, 1996.

Court, William. *Ginseng, The Genus* Panax. Amsterdam: Overseas Publishers Assoc. (CRC Press), 2000.

Diamond, Jared. *Male Menopause*. Naperville, Ill.: Sourcebooks, 1998.

Duke, James. Dr. Duke's Phytochemical and Ethnobotanical Databases, USDA-ARS-NGRL, Beltsville Agricultural Research Center, Beltsville, Md., http://www.ars-grin.gov/cgi-bin/duke/.

———. *The Green Pharmacy*. New York: Rodale Press, 1997.

Felter, Harvey Wickes, and John Uri Lloyd. *King's American Dispensatory*. 2 vols. 1898. Reprint, Sandy, Ore.: Eclectic Medical Publications, 1983.

Foster, Steven. *101 Medicinal Herbs*. Loveland, Colo.: Interweave Press, 1998.

Foster, Steven, and Yue Chongxi. *Herbal Emissaries*. Rochester, Vt.: Healing Arts Press, 1992.

Foster, Steven, and James Duke. *Eastern/Central Medicinal Plants* (Peterson Field Guide). Boston: Houghton Mifflin, 1990.

Fulder, Stephen. *The Book of Ginseng*. Rochester, Vt.: Healing Arts Press, 1993.

Fussell, Betty. *The Story of Corn*. New York: North Point Press, 1999.

Gittleman, Ann Louise. *Super Nutrition for Men*. New York: Avery, 1999.

Gladstar, Rosemary. *Herbal Remedies for Men's Health*. Pownal, Vt.: Storey Books, 1999.

Gladstar, Rosemary, and Pamela Hirsch, eds. *Planting the Future*. Rochester, Vt.: Healing Arts Press, 2000.

Green, James. *The Male Herbal*. Freedom, Calif.: The Crossing Press, 1991.

Greenberg, Beverly. *The DHEA Discovery*. Los Angeles: Majesty Press, 1996.

Harborne, Jeffery, Herbert Baxter, and Gerald P. Moss, eds. *Phytochemical Dictionary: A Handbook of Bioactive Compounds from Plants*. 2nd ed. London: Taylor and Francis, 1999.

Hoffmann, David. *Herbal Prescriptions After 50*. Rev. ed. of *An Elders' Herbal*. Rochester, Vt.: Healing Arts Press, 2007.

———. *The Holistic Herbal*. Rockport, Mass.: Element, 1990.

Kilham, Chris. *Hot Plants*. New York: St. Martins, 2004.

Koch, Heinrich, and Larry Lawson. *Garlic: The Science and Therapeutic Applications of* Allium sativum L. *and Related Species*. Baltimore, Md.: Williams and Wilkins, 1996.

Lenard, Lane. *The Smart Guide to Andro*. Petaluma, Calif.: Smart Publications, 1999.

McClure, Mark. *Smart Medicine for a Healthy Prostate*. New York: Avery, 2000.

Morganthaler, John, and Mia Simms. *The Smart Guide to Better Sex: From Andro to Zinc*. Petaluma, Calif.: Smart Publications, 1999.

Murray, Michael. *Male Sexual Vitality*. Rocklin, Calif.: Prima, 1994.

Murray, Michael, and Joseph Pizzorno. *Encyclopedia of Natural Medicine*. Roseville, Calif.: Prima, 1998.

———. *Textbook of Natural Medicine*. 2nd ed. 2 vols. New York: Churchill Livingstone, 1999.

Nadkarni, K. M. *Indian Materia Medica*. 3rd ed. 2 vols. Bombay: Popular Prakashan, 1954.

Reid, Daniel. *Chinese Herbal Medicine*. Boston: Shambhala, 1986.

Sahelian, Ray. *DHEA: A Practical Guide*. New York: Avery, 1996.

———. *Pregnenolone*. New York: Avery, 1997.

Schuler, Lou. *The Testosterone Advantage Plan*. Emmaus, Pa.: Rodale, 2002.

Schulz, Volker, Rudolf Hänsel, Mark Blumenthal, and V. E. Tyler. *Rational Phytotherapy*. Berlin: Springer, 1998.

Shippen, Eugene, and William Fryer. *The Testosterone Syndrome*. New York: Evans, 1998.

Tan, Robert. *The Andropause Mystery*. Houston: Amred, 2001.

Thijssen, J., and H. Nieuwehnhuyse, eds. *DHEA: A Comprehensive Review*. New York: Parthenon, 1999.

Ullis, Karlis, Joshua Shackman, and Greg Ptacek. *Super T*. New York: Simon and Schuster, 1999.

Walji, Hasnain. *DHEA: The Ultimate Rejuvenating Hormone*. Prescott, Ariz.: Hohm Press, 1996.

Weil, Andrew. *8 Weeks to Optimum Health*. New York: Knopf, 1998.

———. *Spontaneous Healing*. New York: Fawcett Columbine, 1995.

Weiss, Rudolf. *Herbal Medicine*. Gothenberg, Sweden: AB Arcanum, 1988.

Werbach, Melvyn, and Michael Murray. *Biological Influences on Illness*. Tarzana, Calif.: Third Line Press, 1994.

Winston, David. *Saw Palmetto for Men and Women*. North Adams, Mass.: Storey Books, 1999.

Wood, Matthew. *The Book of Herbal Wisdom*. Berkeley, Calif.: North Atlantic Books, 1997.

Wright, Jonathan V., and Lane Lenard. *Maximize Your Vitality and Potency for Men Over 40*. Petaluma, Calif.: Smart Publications, 1999.

Yance, Donald. *Herbal Healing, Medicine, and Cancer*. Chicago: Keats, 1999.

SCIENTIFIC AND POPULAR PAPERS

Disease Conditions

Androgens, Body Mass Index, Weight Studies

Barud, W., et al. "Association of obesity and insulin resistance with serum testosterone, sex hormone binding globulin and estradiol in older males." *Pol Merkuriusz Lek* 19, no. 113 (2005): 634–37.

Castro-Fernandez, C., et al. "A preponderance of circulating basic isoforms is associated with decreased plasma half-life and biological to immunological ration of gonadotropin-releasing hormone, releasable leutenizing hormone in obese men." *J Endocrinol Metab* 85, no. 12 (2000): 4603–10.

Fejes, I., et al. "Effect of body weight on testosterone/estradiol ration in oligozoospermic patients." *Arch Androl* 52, no. 2 (2006): 97–102.

Gapstur, S., et al. "Serum androgen concentrations in young men: A longitudinal analysis of associations with age, obesity, and race; the cardia male hormone study." *Cancer Epidemiology Biomarkers and Prevention* 11 (2002): 1041–47.

Jensen, T. K., et al. "Body mass index in relation to semen quality and reproductive hormones among 1,558 Danish Men." *Fertil Steril* 82, no. 4 (2004): 863–70.

Lima, N., et al. "Decreased androgen levels in massively obese men may be associated with impaired function of the gonadostat." *Int J Obes Relat Metab Disorg* 24, no. 11 (2000): 1433–37.

Pasquali, R. "Obesity and androgens: facts and perspectives." *Fertil Steril* 85, no. 5 (2006): 1319–40.

Pasquali, R., et al. "Adrenal and gonadal function in obesity." *J Endocrinol Invest* 25, no. 10 (2000): 893–98.

Seftel, A. D. "Male hypogonadism: Part I; epidemiology of hypogonadism." *Int J Impot Res* 18, no. 2 (2006): 115–20.

Strain, G. W., et al. "Sex difference in the effect of obesity on 24-hour mean serum gonadotropin levels." *Horm Metab Res* 35, no. 6 (2003): 362–66.

Winters, S. J., et al. "Inhibin-B levels in healthy young adult men and prepubertal boys: Is obesity the cause for the contemporary decline in sperm count because of fewer *Sertoli* cells?" *J Androl,* preprint: http://www.andrology-journal.org/cgi/content/abstract/27/4/560.

Yang, A. J., et al. "Effects on development of the testicle in diet-induced obesity rats." *Wei Shen Yan Jiu* 34, no. 4 (2005): 477–79.

Benign Prostatic Hyperplasia

Cote, R. J., et al. "The effect of finasteride on the prostate gland in men with elevated serum prostate-specific antigen levels." *Br J Cancer* 78 (1998): 413–18.

Ehara, H., et al. "Expression of estrogen receptor in diseased human prostate assessed by non-radioactive in-situ hybridization and immunohistochemistry." *Prostate* 27, no. 6 (1995): 304–13.

Farnsworth, W. E. "Roles of estrogen and SHBG in prostate physiology." *Prostate* 28, no. 1 (1996): 17–23.

Gann, P. H., et al. "A prospective study of plasma hormone levels, nonhormonal factors, and development of benign prostatic hyperplasia." *Prostate* 26, no. 1 (1995): 40–49.

Janter, S. J., et al. "Comparative rates of androgen production and metabolism in Caucasian subjects." *J Clin Endocrinol Metab* 83, no. 6 (1998): 2104–9.

Konety, B. R., et al. "The role of vitamin D in normal prostate growth and differentiation." *Cell Growth Differ* 7 (1996): 1563–70.

Nakkla, A. M., et al. "Estradiol causes the rapid accumulation of cAMP in human prostate." *Proc Natl Acad Sci USA* 91, no. 12 (1994): 5402–5.

Stone, N. N. "Estrogen formation in human prostatic tissue from patients with and without benign prostatic hyperplasia." *Prostate* 9, no. 4 (1986): 311–18.

Voigt, K. D., and W. Bartsch. "The role of tissue steroids in benign hyperplasia and prostate cancer." *Urologe A* 26, no. 6 (1987): 349–57.

Walsh, P. C., et al. "Tissue content of dihydrotestosterone in human prostatic hyperplasia is not supranormal." *J Clin Invest* 72 (1983): 1772–77.

Yamanaka, H., and S. Honma. "Endocrine environment of benign prostatic hyperplasia: prostate size and volume are correlated with serum estrogen concentration." *Scand J Urol Nephrol* 29, no. 1 (1995): 65–68.

Herbs

Black Cohosh

Seidl, M. M., and D. E. Stewart. "Alternative treatments for menopausal symptoms: A systematic review of scientific and lay literature." *Can Fam Phys* 44 (1998): 1299–1308.

Chinese Dogwood

Jeng, H., et al. "A substance isolated from *Cornus officinalis* enhances the motility of human sperm." *American Journal of Chinese Medicine* 25, no. 3–4 (1997): 301–6.

Peng, Q. L., et al. *"Fructus corni* enhances endothelial cell antioxidant defenses." *Gen Pharmacol* 31 (1988): 221–25.

Corn

Bradbury, J. T. "The rabbit ovulating factor of plant juice." *Am J Physiol* 142 (1944): 487–93.

Curruba, M. O., et al. "Stimulatory effect of a maize diet on sexual behaviour of male rats." *Life Sci* 20 (1977): 159–64.

David's Lily

Feng, Shilan, et al. "Studies on the chemical constituents of the flower of David lily." *Zhongguo Zhongyao Zazhi* 19, no. 10 (1994): 611–12, 639.

Janeczko, Anna, and Andrzej Skoczowski. "Mammalian sex hormones in plants." *Folia Histochemica Et Cytobiologica* 43, no. 2 (2005): 71–79.

Stransky, K., et al. "Unusual alkanes pattern of some plant cuticular waxes." *Collection of Szechoslovak Chemical Communications* 56, no. 5 (1991): 1123–29.

Zhang, J. S., Z. H. Yang, and T. H. Tsao. "The occurrence of estrogens in relation to reproductive processes in flowering plants." *Sex Plant Reprod* 4 (1991): 193–96.

Zhong-han, Y., Y. Tang, and Z. X. Cao. "The changes of steroidal sex hormone-testosterone contents in reproductive organs of *Lilium davidii* Duch." *Chih Wu Hsueh Pao* 36, no. 3 (1994): 215–20.

Echinacea

Mostbeck, A., and M. Studlar. "Experimental studies of a plant extract from *Echinacea purpurea* Moench as an unspecific antibody stimulant with special consideration of the influence on the kidney cortex." *Wien Med Wochenschr* 112 (1962): 259–62.

Eleuthero

Dardymov, I. "Gonadotrophic action of *Eleutherococcus glycosides.*" *Lek Sredstva Dal'nego Vostoka* 11 (1972): 60.

Kuntsman, I. "A study of the gonadotrophic activity of the leaves of *Eleutherococcus senticosus.*" *Lek Sredstva Dal'nego Vostoka* 7 (1966): 129–32.

Mkrtchyan, A., et al. "A phase I clinical study of *Androgrographis paniculata* fixed combination Kan Jang versus ginseng and valerian on the semen quality of healthy subjects." *Phytomedicine* 12, no. 6–7 (2005): 403–7.

Garlic

Kasuga, S., et al. "Recent advances on the nutritional effects associated with the use of garlic as a supplement. Pharmacologic activities of aged garlic extract in comparison with other garlic preparations." *J Nutr* 131, no. 3S (2001): 1180S–84S.

Sodimu, O., et al. "Certain biochemical effects of garlic oil on rats maintained on fat-high cholesterol diet." *Experientia* 40, no. 1 (1984): 78–79.

Ginkgo

Cohen, A. J., and B. Bartlik. "*Ginkgo biloba* for anti-depressant induced sexual dysfunction." *J Sex Marital Ther* 24, no. 2 (1998): 139–43.

Pepe, C., et al. "Video capillaroscopy evaluation of efficacy *Ginkgo biloba* extract with L-arginine and magnesium in the treatment of trophic lesions in patients with Stage 4 peripheral arterial occlusive disease." *Minerva Cardioangiol* 47, no. 6 (1999): 223–30.

Sikora, R. *Ginkgo biloba* extract in the therapy of erectile dysfunction," *J Urol* 141 (1989): 188A.

Sohn M., and R. Sikora. *Gingko biloba* extract in the therapy of erectile dysfunction," *J Sex Educ Ther* 17 (1991): 53–61.

Hops

Damber, J. E., et al. "The acute effect of estrogens on testosterone production appears not to be mediated by testicular estrogen receptors." *Mol Cell Endocr* 31, no. 1 (1983): 105–16.

Moger, W. H. "Direct effects of estrogens on the endocrine function of the mammalian testis." *Can J Physiol Pharmacol* 58, no. 9 (1980): 1011–22.

Namiki, M., et al. "Direct inhibitory effect of estrogen on the human testis in vitro." *Arch Androl* 20, no. 2 (1988): 131–35.

Stammel, W., et al. "Tetrahydroisoquinoline alkaloids mimic direct but not receptor-mediated inhibitory effects of estrogens and phytoestrogens on testicular endocrine function. Possible significance for Leydig cell insufficiency in alcohol addiction." *Life Sci* 49, no. 18 (1991): 1319–29.

Licorice

Armanini, D., et al. "Reduction of serum testosterone in men by licorice." *N Engl J Med* 341, no. 15 (1999): 1158.

Edwards, C. R. W. "Lessons from licorice." *N Engl J Med* 325, no. 17 (1991): 1242–43.

Schambelan, M. "Licorice ingestion and blood pressure regulating hormones." *Steroids* 59, no. 2 (1994): 127–30.

Shepherd, Suzanne. "Plant poisoning, licorice." *eMedicine Journal* 2, no. 4 (2001): 2.

Stewart, P. M., et al. "Mineralocorticoid activity of carbenoxolone: Contrasting effects of carbenoxolone and liquorice on 11-beta-hydroxysteroid dehydrogenase activity." *Clin Sci* 78, no. 1 (1990): 49–54.

Muira Puama

Waynberg, J. "Contributions to the clinical validation of the traditional use of *Ptychopetalum guyanna.*" Paper presented at the First International Congress on Ethnopharmacology, Strasbourg, France, June 5–9, 1990.

Waynberg, J. "Male sexual asthenia: Interest in a traditional plant-derived medication." *Ethnopharmacology*, March 1995.

Nettle Root

Belaiche, P., and O. Lievoux. "Clinical studies on the palliative treatment of prostatic adenoma with extract of *urtica* root." *Phytother Res* 5, no. 6 (1991): 267–69.

Bombardelli, E., and P. Morazzoni. "*Urtica dioica L.*" *Fitoterapia* 68, no. 5 (1997): 387–402.

Dathe, G., and H. Schmid. "Phytotherapy of the benign prostatic hyperplasia (BPH): A double blind study with an extract of *Radicis urticae* (ERU)." *Urologe* 27 (1987): 223–26.

Djulepa, J. "A two year study of prostatic syndrome. The results of a conservative treatment with Bazoton." *Arztl Praxis* 63, no. 7 (1982): 2199–2205.

Fieber, F. "Sonographical observations of the course concerning the influence of the medicamentous therapy of the benign prostatic hyperplasia (BPH)." In *Klinische Und Experimentelle Urologie 19. Benigne Prostathyperplasie II*, edited by H. W. Bower. Napralert database citation (www.napralert.org), 1988: 75–82.

Friesen. A. "Statistical analysis of a multicenter longterm study with ERU1." Napralert citation, 1988: 121–130.

Goetz, P. "Treatment of benign prostatic hyperplasia with *Urticae Radix*." *Z Phytother* 10 (1989): 175–8.

Hartmann, R. W., et al. "Inhibition of 5 alpha-reductase and aromatase by PHL-00801 (Prostatonin), a combination of PY 102 *(Pygeum africanum)* and UR 102 *(Urtica dioica)* extracts." *Phytomedicine* 3, no. 2 (1996): 121–28.

Hryb, D. J., et al. "The effect of extracts of the root of the stinging nettle *(Urtica dioica)* on the interaction of SHBG with its receptor on human prostatic membranes." *Planta Med* 61, no. 1 (1995): 31–32.

Kraus, K., et al. "(10E,12Z)-9-Hydroxy-10,12-Octadecadienoic Acid, an aromatase inhibitor from roots of *Urtica dioica*." *Liebigs Ann Chem* 4 (1991): 335–39.

Krzeski, T., et al. "Combined extracts of *Urtica dioica* and *Pygeum africanum* in the treatment of benign prostatic hyperplasia: double-blind comparison of two doses." *Clin Ther* 15, no. 6 (1993): 1011–20.

Lichius, J. J., and C. Muth. "The inhibiting effects of *Urtica dioica* root extracts on experimentally induced prostatic hyperplasia in the mouse." *Planta Med* 63, no. 4 (1997): 307–10.

Lichius, J. J., et al. "The inhibiting effects of components of stinging nettle roots on experimentally induced prostatic hyperplasia in mice." *Planta Med* 65, no. 7 (1999): 666–68.

Lowe, F. C., and E. Fagelman. "Phytotherapy in the treatment of benign prostatic hyperplasia: an update." *Urology* 53, no. 4 (1999): 671–78.

Lowe, F. C., et al. "Review of recent placebo-controlled trials utilizing phytotherapeutic agents for the treatment of BPH." *Prostate* 37, no. 3 (1998): 187–93.

Maar, K. "Retrogression of the symptomatology of prostate adenoma. Results of a six months conservative treatment with ERU capsules." *Fortschr Med* 105 (1987): 1–5.

Montanari, E., et al. "Benign prostatic hyperplasia randomized study with 63 patients." *Informierte Arzt* 6A (1991): 593–98.

Oberholzer, M., et al. "Results obtained by electron microscopy in medicamentously treated benign prostatic hyperplasia (BPH)." In *Benigne Prostatahyperplasie*, edited by H. W. Bauer. Napralert citation, 1986: 13–17.

Romics, I. "Observations with Bazoton in the management of prostatic hyperplasia." *Int Urol Nephrol* 19, no. 3 (1987): 293–97.

Schmidt, K. "The effect of an extract of *Radix Urticae* and various secondary extracts on the SHBG of blood plasma in benign prostatic hyperplasia." *Fortschr Med* 101, no. 21 (1983): 713–16.

Schottner, Matthias, Gerhard Spireller, and Dietmar Gansser. "Lignans interfering with 5a-dihydrotestosterone binding to human sex hormone-binding globulin." *J Nat Prod* 61 (1998): 119–21.

Stahl, H. P. "Therapy of prostatic nocturia with a standardized extract of *urtica* root." *Z Allg Med* 60 (1984): 128–32.

Suh, N., et al. "Discovery of natural product chemopreventative agents utilizing HL-60 cell differentiation as a model." *Anticancer Res* 15, no. 2 (1995): 233–39.

Tosch, U., and H. Mussiggang. "The Medicamentous treatment of the benign prostatic hyperplasia." *Euromed* 6 (1983): 1–8.

Vahlensieck, W. "Konservative behandling der benign prostathyperplasie (BPH)." *Therapiewoche* 35 (1985): 4031–40.

Vontobel, H. P., et al. "The results of a double-blind study on the efficacy of ERU capsules in the conservative treatment of benign prostatic hyperplasia." *Urologe* 24 (1985): 49–51.

Wagner, H., et al. "Biologically active compounds from the aqueous extract of *Urtica dioica*." *Planta Med* 55, no. 5 (1989): 452–54.

Wagner, H., et al. "Search for the antiprostatic principle of stinging nettle *(Urtica dioica)* roots." *Phytomedicine* 1, no. 3 (1994): 213–24.

Zieglar, H. "Investigations of prostate cells under effect of extract *Radix Urticae* (ERU) by fluorescent microscopy." *Fortschr Med* 45 (1983): 2112–14.

Ziegler, V. H. "Zytomorphologische verlaufskontrolle einer therapie der residivierenden prostatis durch eine landzeit-kombinations behandlung." *Fortschr Med* 39, no. 21 (1982): 1832–34.

Oats

Bradbury, J. T. "The rabbit ovulating factor of plant juice." *Am J Physiol* 142 (1944): 487–93.

Panax ginseng

Note: the National Library of Medicine's PubMed Medline online database (www.ncbi.nlm.nih.gov/entrez/) lists 2,530 studies as of June 1, 2006, and this does not include the hundreds or thousands more not yet translated from Chinese journals. The journal citations in the following consulted sources are only a sample. Extensive resource material is present in the texts listed in the general bibliography.

Chen, Q. H., et al. "Pharmacology of total saponins of the fibrous roots of *Panax notoginseng.*" *Chung Yao T'ung Pao* 12, no. 3 (1987): 173–75.

Fahim, M. S., et al. Effect of *Panax ginseng* on testosterone level and prostate in male rats." *Arch Androl* 8 (1982): 261–63.

Ge, Ry, and H. Pu. "Effects of ginsenosides and pantocrine on the reproductive endocrine system in male rats." *J Trad Chin Med* 6, no. 4 (1986): 301–4.

Popov, I. M., and C. F. Hering III. "The use of ginseng extract as an adjunct in different types of treatment for male impotency." *Abstr Third Int Ginseng Symp Korea*, Res Inst, Soul, Korea, Sept. 8–10, 1980, p. 10.

Salvati, G., et al. "Effects of *Panax ginseng* C. A. Meyer saponins on male fertility." *Panminerva Med* 38, no. 4 (1996): 249–54.

Tsai, S. C., et al. "Stimulation of the secretion of luteinizing hormone by ginsenoside-Rb1 in male rats." *Chin J Physiol* 46, no. 1 (2003): 1–7.

Wang, J., et al. "Experimental research on the regulating effects of ginseng with hairy antler on the sexual dysfunction rat model induced with adenine." *Zhonghua Nan Ke Xue* 10, no. 4 (2004): 315–19.

Youl, Kang H., et al. "Effects of ginseng ingestion on growth hormone, testosterone, cortisol, and insulin-like growth factor 1 responses to acute resistance exercise." *Journal of Strength and Conditioning Research* 16, no. 2 (2002): 179–83.

Pine Pollen

Armentia, A., et al. "Allergy to pine pollen and pinon nuts: A review of three cases; Comment." *Ann Allergy* 64, no. 5 (1990): 480.

Fan, Bo-Lin, et al. "Toxicological Research of Pollen Pini." Abstract. Chinese Electronic Periodicals Service (CEPS), catalog number 203581, 2005.

Freeman, G. "Pine pollen allergy in northern Arizona." *Ann Allergy* 60, no. 6 (1993): 491–94.

Garcia, J. J., et al. "Pollinosis due to Australian pine *(Casuarina)*: An aerobiologic and clinical study in southern Spain." *Allergy* 52, no. 1 (1997): 11–17.

Hanssen, Maurice. *The Healing Power of Pollen.* Wellingborough, Northhamptonshire, U.K.: Thorsons, 1979. Appendix: "A Comparative Analysis of Three Pollens: *Zea Mays, Alnus spp.,* and *Pinus Montana.* www.graminex.com.

Harris, R., and D. German. "The incidence of pine pollen reactivity in an allergic atopic population." *Ann Allergy* 55, no. 5 (1985): 678–79.

Helmers, H., and L. Machlis. "Exogenous substrate utilization and fermentation by the pollen of *Pinus ponderosa.*" *Plant Physiology* 31, no. 4 (1956): 284–89.

Janeczko, Anna, and Andrzej Skoczowski. "Mammalian sex hormones in plants." *Folia Histochemica Et Cytobiologica* 43, no. 2 (2005): 71–79.

Jenkins, Ronald, et al. "Androstendione and progesterone in the sediment of a river receiving paper mill effluent." *Toxicological Sciences* 73, no. 1 (2003): 53–59.

———. "Identification of androstenedione in a river containing paper mill effluent." *Environmental Toxicology and Chemistry* 20, no. 6 (2001): 1325–31.

Kalliel, J., and G. Settipane. "Eastern pine sensitivity in New England." *N Engl Reg Allergy Proc* 9, no. 3 (1988): 233–35.

Kamienska, A., and R. Pharis. "Endogenous gibberellins of pine pollen: II. Changes during germination of *Pinus attenuata, P. coulteri,* and *P. ponderosa* pollen." *Plant Physiology* 56, no. 5 (1975): 655–59.

Kamienska, A., R. Durley, and R. Pharis. "Endogenous gibberellins of pine pollen: III. Conversion of 1,2-[H]GA(4) to gibberellins A(1) and A(34) in germinating pollen of *Pinus attenuata* Lemm." *Plant Physiology* 58, no. 1 (1976): 68–70.

Kim, Song-Ki, et al. "Identification of two brassinosteroids from the cambial region of Scots pine *(Pinus silvestris)* by gas chromoatography-mass spectrometry, after deteching using a dwarf rice lamina inclination bioassay." *Plant Physiol* 94 (1990): 1709–13.

Lee, Eun Ju, and Thomas Booth. "Macronutrient input from pollen in two regenerating pine stands in southeast Korea." *Ecological Research* 18, no. 4 (2003): 423–30.

Ma, Y. "Determination of amino acids in pollen of *Pinus tabulaeformis* by pico tag method." *Chinese Journal of Chromatography* 12, no. 1 (1994): 63.

Marcos, C., et al. "*Pinus* pollen aerobiology and clinical sensitization in northwest Spain." *Ann Allergy Asthma Immunol* 87, no. 1 (2001): 39–42.

Oleksyn, J., et al. "Nutritional status of pollen and needles of diverse *Pinus sylvestris* populations grown at sites with contrasting pollution." *Water, Air, and Soil Pollution* 110, no. 1–2 (1999): 195–212.

Parks, L., et al. "Masculinization of female mosquitofish in Kraft mill effluent-contaminated Fenholloway river water is associated with androgen receptor agonist activity." *Toxicological Sciences* 62, no. 2 (2001): 257–67.

Saden-Krehula, M., and M. Tajic. "Vitamin D and its metabolites in the pollen of pine. Part 5: Steroid hormones in the pollen of pine species." *Pharmazie* 42, no. 7 (1987): 471–72.

Saden-Krehula, M., M. Tajic, and D. Kolbah. "Sex hormones and corticosteroids in pollen of *Pinus nigra*." *Phytochemistry* 17 (1978): 345–46.

Saden-Krehula, M., et al. "Steroid hormones in the pollen of pine species IV.: 17-ketosteroids in *Pinus nigra* Ar." *Naturwissenschaften* 70, no. 10 (1983): 520–22.

Saden-Krehula, M., et al. "Testosterone, epitestosterone, and androstenedione in the pollen of scotch pine, *Pinus sylvestris* L." *Experientia* 27 (1971): 108–9.

Senna, G., et al. "Anaphylaxis to pine nuts and immunological cross-reactivity with pine pollen proteins." *J Investig Allergol Clin Immunol* 10, no. 1 (2000): 44–46.

Wang, Ting, et al. "Provitamins and vitamin D2 and D3 in *Cladina* spp. over a latitudinal gradient: possible correlation with UV levels." *Journal of Photochemistry and Photobiology, B-Biology* 62 (2001): 118–22.

Wang, Y., H. J. Wang, and Z. Y. Zhang. "Analysis of pine pollen by using FTIR, SEM, and energy-dispersive X-ray analysis." *Guang Pu Xue Yu Guang Pu Fen Xi* 25, no. 11 (2005): 1797–800.

Zeng, Qing-Yin, Hai Lu, and Xiao-Ru Wang. "Molecular characterization of a glutathione transferase from *Pinus tabulaeformis* (Pinaceae)." *Biochimie* 87 (2005): 445–55.

Zhao, L., W. Windisch, and M. Kirchgessner. "A study on the nutritive value of pollen from the Chinese masson pine *(Pinus massoniana)* and its effect on fecal characteristics in rats." *Z Ernahrungswiss* 35, no. 4 (1996): 341–47.

Zhi, Chong-Yuan, and Kai-Fa Wang. "A study on nutrient components of pollen grains of *Pinus tabulaeformis, Pinus bungeana,* and *Picea wilsonii.*" Abstract. Chinese electronic Periodicals Service (CEPS), catalog number 228270, 2001.

Pine Nuts

Note: General information about pine nuts can be found at the following Web sites:

http://www.birdways.com
http://www.medicalmeals.com
http://www.nat.uiuc.edu
http://www.vegsoc.org

Gutierrez-Fernandez, M. R., et al., "Methods for the study of estrone, estradiol and testosterone in the seeds of *Pinus pinea* L." *An R Acad Farm* 47, no. 1 (1981): 97–112.

Rye Grass Pollen

Buck, A. C., et al. "Treatment of outflow tract obstruction due to benign prostatic hyperplasia with the pollen extract, Cernilton: A double-blind, placebo-controlled Study." *Br J Urol* 66, no. 4 (1990): 398–404.

Habib, F. K., et al. "In vitro evaluation of the pollen extract, Cernitin T-60, in the regulation of prostate cell growth." *Br J Urol* 66, no. 4 (1990): 393–7.

Jodai, A., et al. "A long-term therapeutic experience with Cernilton in chronic prostatitis." *Hinyokika Kiyo* 34 (1988): 561–68.

Rugendorff, E. W., et al, "Results of treatment with pollen extract (Cernilton N) in chronic prostatitis and prostatodynia." *Br J Urol* 71 (1993): 433–38.

Wojcicki, J., et al. "Effect of flower pollen in patients with rheumatoid arthritis and concomitant diseases of the gastroduodenal and hepatobiliary systems." *Likarska Sprava* 4 (1998): 151–54.

Yasumoto, R., et al. "Clinical evaluation of long-term treatment using Cernilton pollen extract in patients with benign prostatic hyperplasia." *Clinical Therapeutics* 17 (1995): 82–86.

Saw Palmetto

Awang, D. V. C. "Saw palmetto, African prune, and stinging nettle for benign prostatic hyperplasia (BPH)." *Can Pharm J* 130, no. 9 (1997): 37–44–62.

Braeckman, J. "The extract of *Serenoa repens* in the treatment of benign prostatic hyperplasia: A multicenter open study." *Curr Ther Res* 55 (1994): 776–85.

Braeckman, J., et al. "Efficacy and safety of the extract of *Serenoa repens* in the treatment of benign prostatic hyperplasia." *Phytotherapy Research* 11 (1997): 558–63.

Broccafoschi, S., and S. Amnoscia. "Comparison of *Serenoa repens* extract with placebo in controlled clinical trial in patients with prostatic adenomatosis." *Urologia* 50 (1983): 1257–68.

Caponera, M., et al. "Antiestrogenic activity of *Serenoa repens* in patients with BPH." *Acta Urol Ital* 6, suppl. 4 (1992): 271–72.

Champault, G., et al. "Medical treatment of prostatic adenoma: Controlled trial; PA 109 vs. placebo in 110 patients." *Ann Urol* 18 (1984): 4–7, 10.

Di Silverio, F., et al. "Effects of long-term treatment with *Serenoa repens* (Permixon) on the concentrations and regional distribution of androgens and epidermal growth factor in benign prostatic hyperplasia." *Prostate* 37, no. 2 (1992): 77–83.

———. "Evidence that *Serenoa repens* extract displays an antiestrogenic activity in prostatic tissue of benign prostatic hypertrophy patients." *Eur Urol* 21, no. 4 (1992): 309–14.

Koch, E. "Pharmacology and modes of action of extracts of palmetto fruit *(Sabal fructus)*, stinging nettle roots *(Urticae radix)*, and pumpkin seed *(Curcurbitae peponis semen)* in the treatment of benign prostatic hyperplasia." *Phytopharmaka forsch Klin Anwend* (1995): 57–79.

Koch, E., and A. Biber. "Pharmacological effects of saw palmetto and *urtica* extracts for benign prostatic hyperplasia." *Quart Rev Nat Med* (1995): 281–289.

Marks, L. S., et al. "Effects of a saw palmetto herbal blend in men with symptomatic benign prostatic hyperplasia." *J Urol* 163, no. 5 (2000): 1451–56.

———. "Tissue effects of saw palmetto and Finasteride: use of biopsy cores for in situ quantification of prostatic androgens." *Urology* 57, no. 5 (2001): 999–1005.

McKinney, D. E. "Saw palmetto for benign prostatic hyperplasia." *J Amer Med Ass* 281, no. 18 (1999): 1699.

Schneider, H. J., et al. "Treatment of benign prostatic hyperplasia. Results of a surveillance study in the practices of urological specialists using a combined plant-based preparation (*Sabal* extract WS 1473 and *urtica* extract WS 1031)." *Fortschr Med* 113, no. 3 (1995): 37–40.

Stokeland, J. "Combined *Sabal* and *Urtica* extract compared with Finasteride in men with benign prostatic hyperplasia: an analysis of prostate volume and therapeutic outcome." *Brit J Urol Int* 86, no. 4 (2000): 439–42.

Stokeland, J., and J. Albrecht. "Combined *Sabal* and *urtica* extract vs. Finasteride in BPH (Alken Stage I–II)." *Urology* 36 (1997): 327–33.

Strauch, G., et al. "Comparison of finasteride (Proscar) and *Serenoa repens* in the inhibition of 5-alpha reductase in healthy male volunteers." *Eur Urol* 26, no. 3 (1994): 247–52.

Vahlensieck, W., Jr., et al. Benign prostatic hyperplasia: Treatment with sabal fruit extract." *Fortschritte Med* 111 (1993): 323–26.

Speman

Agarway, V. K., and R. K. Gupta. "Clinical studies with speman in cases of benign enlargement of the prostate." *The Indian Practitioner* 6 (1971): 281.

Ahmed, Mir Nazir, et al. "Speman in patients of benign prostatomegaly." *Current Medical Practice* 9 (1983): 257.

Bannerjee, P. "Speman and cystone in benign prostatic enlargement." *Probe* 13, no. 2 (1974): 88–90.

Gaur, K. P. "Evaluation of speman in prostatitis." *Capsule* 1 (1982): 2.

Gour, K. N., and Sudhir Gupta. "Speman in male sexual disorders." *Current Medical Practice* 3 (1959): 135.

Jayatilak, P. G., et al. "Effect of an indigenous drug (Speman) on human accessory reproductive function." *Indian J Surg* 38 (1976): 12–15.

———. "Effect of an indigenous drug (Speman) on accessory reproduction functions in mice." *Indian J Exp Biol* 14 (1976): 170.

Limaye, H. R., and C. S. Madkar. "Management of oligozoospermia, asthenospermia, and necrozoospermia by treatment with 'Speman.'" *Antiseptic* (1984): 612.

Madaan, S., and T. R. Madaan. "Speman in oligospermia." *Probe* 24, no. 2 (1985): 115–17.

Mukher, S., et al. "Effect of Speman on prostatism: A clinical study." *Probe* 25 (1986): 237–40.

Pardanani, D. S., et al. "Study of the effects of speman on semen quality in oligospermic men." *Indian J Surg* 38 (1976): 34–39.

Rathore, H. S., and V. Saraswat. "Protection of mouse testes, epididymis, and adrenals with speman against cadmium intoxication." *Probe* 25 (1986): 257–68.

Sengupta, Sabuj. "A clinico-pathological study of the effect of Speman on spermatogenesis in cases of oligozoospermia." *Probe* 21, no. 4 (1982): 275–76.

Tienchi Ginseng

Note: Research is becoming significant; the National Library of Medicine's PubMed Medline online database (www.ncbi.nlm.nih.gov/entrez/) lists 239 citations as of June 1, 2006. There are hundreds more in Chinese databases that have not yet been translated. The following articles on tienchi ginseng are only a sample of those available that were consulted in writing this book.

Chan, Robbie Y. K., et al. "Estrogen-like activity of ginsenoside Rg1 derived from *Panax notoginseng*." *The Journal of Clinical Endocrinology and Metabolism* 87, no. 8 (2002): 3691–95.

Chen, J. C., et al. "Effects of ginsenoside Rb2 and Re on inferior human sperm motility in vitro." *Am J Chin Med* 29, no. 1 (2001): 155–60.

———. "Effect of *panax notoginseng* extracts on inferior sperm motility in vitro." *Am J Chin Med* 27, no. 1 (1999): 123–28.

———. "Effects of *Panax notoginseng* polysaccharide and aqueous fraction on human sperm motility in vitro." *China Med Coll J* 7, no. 4 (1998): 39–46.

———. Effect of *Panax notoginseng* saponins on sperm motility and progression in vitro." *Phytomedicine* 5, no. 4 (1998): 289–92.

Chen, Q. H., et al. "Pharmacology of the total saponins of the fibrous roots of *Panax notoginseng*." *Chung Yao T'ung Pao* [Chinese Journal of Chinese Materia Medica] 12, no. 3 (1987): 173–75.

Gao, H., et al. "Immunomodulating polysaccharides from *Panax notoginseng*." *Pharm Res* 13, no. 8 (1996): 1196–1200.

He, W., and Z. Zhu. "Effect of *Panax notoginseng* saponins on intercellular adhesion molecule-I expression and neutrophil infiltration in cerebral infarction tissue of rats." *Zhong Yao Cai* 28, no. 5 (2005): 403–5.

Liang, M. T., T. D. Podolka, and W. J. Chuang. "*Panax notoginseng* supplementation enhances physical performance during endurance exercise." *J Strength Cond Res* 19, no. 1 (2005): 108–14.

Shi, Qin, et al. "Ginsenoside Rd from *Panax notoginseng* enhances astrocyte differentiation from neural stem cells." *Life Sci* 76 (2005): 983–95.

Wu, Y., et al. "The pharmacokinetics and pharmacodynamics on intranasal preparations of *Panax notoginseng* saponins." *Yao Xue Xue Bao* 40, no. 4 (2005): 377–81.

Yang, B. H., et al. "Effects of *Astragalus membranaceus* and *Panax notoginseng* on the transformation of bone marrow stem cells and the proliferation of EPC in vitro." *Zhongguo Zhong Yao Za Zhi* 30, no. 22 (2005): 1761–63.

Zhang, Hong, et al. "Ginsenoside Re increases fertile and asthenozoospermic infertile human sperm motility by induction of nitric oxide synthase." *Arch Pharm Res* 29, no. 2 (2006): 145–51.

Zhong, Z., et al. "Effects of the *Panax notoginseng* saponins on the level of synaptophysin protein in brain in rat model with lesion of Meynert." *Zhongguo Zhong Yao Za Zhi* 30, no. 12 (2005): 913–15.

Zhu, Y., et al. "Characterization of cell wall polysaccharides from the medicinal plant *Panax notoginseng.*" *Phytochemistry* 66, no. 9 (2005): 1067–76.

Tribulus

Note: Extensive research sources are available online at http://www.libolov.com and http://www.tribestan.com. The following material is representative.

Adaikan, P. G., K. Gauthaman, and R. Prasad. "History of herbal medicines with an insight on the pharmacological properties of *Tribulus terrestris.*" *Aging Male* 4, no. 3 (2001): 163–69.

Adaikan, P. G., et al. "Proerectile pharmacological effects of *Tribulus terrestris* extract on the rabbit corpus cavernosum." *Ann Acad Med Singapore* 29, no. 1 (2000): 22–26.

Adimoelja, A. "Phytochemicals and the breakthrough of traditional herbs in the management of sexual dysfunction." *Int J Androl* 23, no. 2 (2000): 82–84.

———. "Treatment of Sexual dysfunction in diabetes mellitus subjects using orally administered protodioscin and injection of vasoactive compounds." Proceedings from the Seminar of Erectile Dysfunction of Diabetes, Bandung, Indonesia, 1997.

Adimoelja, A., and P. Ganeshan Adaikan. "Protodioscin from herbal plant *Tribulus terrestris* improves the male sexual functions, probably via DHEA." *Int J Impotence Research* 9, no. 1 (1997): S64.

Arsyad, K. M. "Effect of protodioscin on the quantity and quality of sperms from males with moderate oligozoospermia." *Medika* 22, no. 8 (1996): 614–18.

Gauthaman, K., and P. Adaikan. "Effect of *Tribulus terrestris* on nicotinamide adenine dinucleotide phosphate-diaphorase activity and androgen receptors in rat brain." *J Ethnopharmacol* 96, no. 1–2 (2005): 127–32.

Gauthaman, K., P. Adaikan, and R. Prasad. "Aphrodisiac properties of *Tribulus terrestris* extract (Ptotodioscin) in normal and castrated rats." *Life Sci* 71, no. 12 (2002): 1385–96.

Gauthaman, K., A. Ganasan, and R. Prasad. "Sexual effects of puncturevine *(Tribulus terrestris)* extract (protodioscin): an evaluation using a rat model." *J Altern Complement Med* 9, no. 2 (2003): 257–65.

Gauthaman, K., et al. "Changes in hormonal parameters secondary to intravenous administration of *Tribulus terrestris* extract in primates." *International Journal of Impotence Research* 12, supplement 6 (2000): 6.

———. "Pro-erectile pharmacological effect of *Tribulis terrestris* on the rabbit corpus cavernosum." *Ann Acad Med Singapore* 29, no. 1 (2000): 22–26.

Kaumanov, F., et al. "Clinical trial of Tribestan." *Experimental Medicine* 2 (1982): 8.

Milanov, S., et al. "Tribestan effect on the concentration of some hormones in the serum of healthy subjects." http://www.tribestan.com.

Moeloek, N., et al. "Trials of *Tribulus terrestris* (Protodioscin) on Oligozoospermia." Proceedings of the Sixth National Congress and Third International Symposium on New Perspectives of Andrology on Human Reproduction, 1994. http://www.tribestan.com.

Nasution, A. W. "Effect of *Tribulus terrestris* treatment on impotence and libido disorders." Andalas University School of Medicine. http://www.liboliv.com (accessed June 1, 2006).

Obreshkova, D., et al. "Comparative analytical investigation of *Tribulus terrestris* preparations." *Pharmacia* 15, no. 2 (1998): 11.

Pangkahila, W. "*Tribulus terrestris* (Protodioscin) Increases Men's Sex Drive." Proceedings of the Tenth National Congress on New Perspectives of Andrology on Human Reproduction. http://www.pharmabul.com/research.htm (accessed June 1, 2006).

Sankaran, J. "Problem of male virility: An oriental therapy." *J Natl Integ Med Assoc* 26, no. 11 (1984): 315–17.

Setiawan, L. "*Tribulus terrestris* L. extract improves spermatozoa motility and increases the efficiency of acrosome reaction in subjects diagnosed with oligoasthenoteratozoospermia." *J Panca Sarjana Aialangga University 5*, no. 2–3 (1996): 35–40.

Tomova, M., et al. "Steroidal saponins from *Tribulus terristris* with a stimulating action on the sexual functions." *Int Conf Chem Biotenhnol Biol Act Nat Prod* 3 (1981): 298–302.

Viktorof, I., et al. "Pharmacological, pharmacokinetic, toxicological and clinical studies on protodioscin." *IIMS Therapeutic Focus* 2 (1994). http://www.nutrica.com/Libilov/LMR1.htm (accessed June 1, 2006).

Nutritional Supplements

L-arginine

Keller, D. W., and K. L. Polakoski. "L-arginine stimulation of human sperm motility in vitro." *Biol Reprod* 13 (1975): 154–57.

Pearson, Durk, and Sandy Shaw. "Sexual effects of nutrients: arginine and choline." *Lifenet News* 2 (1999): 6.

Schacter, A., J. A. Goldman, and Z. Zuckerman. "Treatment of Oligospermia with the Amino Acid Arginine." *J Urol* 110 (1973): 311–13.

Yoram, V., and G. Illan. "Oral pharmacotherapy in erectile dysfunction." *Curr Opin Urol* 7, no. 6 (1997): 349–53.

Zorgniotti, A. W., and E. F. Lia. "Effect of large doses of nitric oxide precursor, L-arginine, on erectile dysfunction." *Int J Impot Rev* 1 (1994): 33–35.

L-carnitine

Vitali, G., R. Parente, and C. Melotti. "Carnitine supplementation in Human Idiopathic Asthenospermia: Clinical results." *Drugs Exp Clin Res* 21 (1995): 157–59.

L-choline

Yoram, V., and G. Illan. "Oral pharmacotherapy in erectile dysfunction." *Curr Opin Urol* 7, no. 6 (1997): 349–53.

Zorgniotti, A. W., and E. F. Lia. "Effect of large doses of nitric oxide precursor, L-arginine, on erectile dysfunction." *Int J Impot Rev* 1 (1994): 33–35.

DHT

Arnold, Patrick. "DHT: Is It All Bad?" Reprinted from *Muscle Monthly Magazine*. http://ww.mesomorphosis.com/articles/arnold.dht.htm.

Avila, D. M., et al. "Identification of genes expressed in the rat prostate that are modulated differently by castration and finasteride treatment." *Journal of Endocrinology* 159 (1996): 403–11.

Endocrine Society. "Dihydrotestosterone Gel Increases Muscle, Decreases Fat in Older Men." September 14, 2001, Press Release, reporting on the results of a study conducted at the University of Sydney and published in the September 2001 issue of the *Journal of Clinical Endocrinology and Metabolism* (2001).

Llewellyn, William. "DHT and the Athlete: Is It the Enemy?" http://www.hon-online.com/dht.html.

Negri-Cesi, P., et al. "Metabolism of steroids in the brain: A new insight into the role of 5alpha-reductase and aromatase in brain differentiation and functions." *J. Steroid Biochem Mol Biol* 58 (1996): 455–66.

Poletti, A., and L. Martini. "Androgen-activating enzymes in the central nervous system." *J Steroid Biochem Mol Biol* 65 (1998): 295–99.

Poletti, A., et al. "The 5 alpha-reductase isozymes in the central nervous system." *Steroids* 63 (1998): 246–51.

L-pherylalanine and L-tryrosine

Yoram, V., and G. Illan. "Oral pharmacotherapy in erectile dysfunction." *Curr Opin Urol* 7, no. 6 (1997): 349–53.

Omega-3 Fatty Acids

Hart, J., and W. Cooper. *Vitamin F in the Treatment of Prostatic Hypertrophy.* Milwaukee, Wis.: Lee Foundation for Nutritional Research, 1941.

Lanier, A. P., et al. "Cancer in Alaskan Indians, Eskimos, and Aleuts, 1969–1983: Implications for etiology and control." *Public Health Rep* 27 (1989): 798–803.

Vitamin B

Kumamato, Y., et al. "Clinical efficacy of mecobalamin in treatment of oligospermia: Results of a double-blind comparative clinical study." *Acta Urol Japan* 34 (1988): 1109–32.

Sandler, B., and B. Faragher. "Treatment of oligospermia with Vitamin B12." *Infertility* 7 (1984): 133–38.

Zinc

Netter, A., et al. "Effect of zinc administration on plasma testosterone, dihydrotestosterone, and sperm count." *Arch Androl* 7 (1981): 69–73.

Tikkiwal, M. "Effect of zinc administration on seminal zinc and fertility of oligospermic males." *Ind Journal Physiol Pharmacol* 31 (1987): 30–34.

Foods

Alcohol

Derosa, G., et al. "Prolactin secretion after beer." *Lancet* 2 (1981): 934.

Stammel, W., et al. "Tetrahydroisoquinoline alkaloids mimic direct but not receptor-mediated inhibitory effects of estrogens and phytoestrogens on testicular endocrine function. Possible significance for Leydig cell insufficiency in alcohol addiction." *Life Sci* 49, no. 18 (1991): 1319–29.

Tazuke, S., et al. "Exogenous estrogen and endogenous sex hormones." *Medicine* 71 (1992): 44–50.

Meat

Hamalainen, E., et al. "Diet and serum sex hormones in healthy men." *J Steroid Biochem* 20 (1984): 459–64.

INDEX